C000099896

Parkinsonian Disorders in Clinical Practice

Supported by an educational grant from Boehringer Ingelheim International GmbH

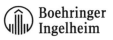 Boehringer Ingelheim

Editorial coordination and management: Armine Najand, MD, Daniel Beard

LMS Group
75 rue Guy Môquet
92240 Malakoff
France
Phone: +33 1 42 53 03 03
Fax: +33 1 42 53 03 02
E-mail: info@lms-group.com
www.lms-group.com

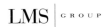

Parkinsonian Disorders in Clinical Practice

EDITED BY

Anthony H.V. Schapira MD, DSc
FRCP, FMedSci

Head of Department, University Department of Clinical Neurosciences,
Institute of Neurology, Queen Square, London, UK
Professor of Neurology, National Hospital for Neurology and Neurosurgery,
and Royal Free Hospital, London, UK

Andreas Hartmann MD

Clinical Investigation Center, Pitié-Salpêtrière Hospital, Paris, France
Federation of Nervous System Diseases, Pitié-Salpêtrière Hospital, Paris, France
National Institute of Health and Medical Research (INSERM U679), Paris, France
Pierre and Marie Curie University, Paris, France

Yves Agid MD, PhD

Clinical Investigation Center, Pitié-Salpêtrière Hospital, Paris, France
Federation of Nervous System Diseases, Pitié-Salpêtrière Hospital, Paris, France
National Institute of Health and Medical Research (INSERM U679), Paris, France
Pierre and Marie Curie University, Paris, France

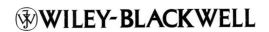

ISBN: 978-1-4051-8405-2

A catalogue record for this book is available from the British Library.

Set in 9.5/12pt Palatino by Sparks, Oxford – www.sparkspublishing.com

Printed and bound in Singapore by Utopia Press Pte Ltd

First published 2008

1 2008

Contents

List of contributors

Yves Agid MD, PhD
Clinical Investigation Center, Pitié-Salpêtrière
Hospital; Federation of Nervous System Diseases,
Pitié-Salpêtrière Hospital; National Institute of
Health and Medical Research (INSERM U679);
Pierre et Marie Curie University, Paris, France

Kailash P. Bhatia MD
Sobell Department of Motor Neuroscience and
Movement Disorders, Institute of Neurology,
University College London, National Hospital
for Neurology and Neurosurgery, Queen Square,
London, UK

Alexis Brice MD
Pierre et Marie Curie University, Pitié-Salpêtrière
Medical School; Federative Institute for
Neuroscience Research; Department of Genetics
and Cytogenetics, Federation of Nervous System
Diseases, Pitié-Salpêtrière Hospital, Paris, France

Perrine Charles MD, PhD
Pierre et Marie Curie University, Pitié-Salpêtrière
Medical School; Federative Institute for
Neuroscience Research; Department of Genetics
and Cytogenetics, Federation of Nervous System
Diseases, Pitié-Salpêtrière Hospital, Paris, France

Yaroslau Compta MD
Parkinson's Disease and Movement
Disorders Unit, Neurology Service, Institut
Clínic de Neurociències, Hospital Clínic de
Barcelona, Universitat de Barcelona, Institut
d'Investigacions Biomèdiques August Pi I Sunyer
(IDIBAPS), Centro de Investigación Biomédica
en Red sobre Enfermedades Neurodegenerativas
(CIBERNED), Barcelona, Spain

Virginie Czernecki PhD
Behavioral Unit and Federation of Neurology;
Pitié-Salpêtrière Hospital; Pierre et Marie Curie
University Paris VI, Paris, France

Philippe Damier MD, PhD
CHU Nantes, Clinique Neurologique and Centre
d'Investigation Clinique, Nantes, France

Ruth Djaldetti MD
Department of Neurology, Rabin Medical
Center, Beilinson Campus, Petah Tiqwa, and
Sackler Faculty of Medicine, Tel Aviv University,
Tel Aviv, Israel

Bruno Dubois MD, PhD
Behavioral Unit and Federation of Neurology;
Pitie-Salpetriere Hospital; Pierre et Marie Curie
University Paris VI, Paris, France

Alexandra Dürr MD, PhD
Pierre et Marie Curie University; Federative
Institute for Neuroscience Research (IFR70);
Department of Genetics and Cytogenetics,
Pitié-Salpêtrière Hospital, Paris, France

Murat Emre MD
Professor of Neurology, Istanbul University,
Istanbul Faculty of Medicine, Department
of Neurology, Behavioral Neurology and
Movement Disorders Unit, Çapa Istanbul, Turkey

Leorah Freeman MD
Department of Genetics and Cytogenetics, Pitié-
Salpêtrière Hospital, Paris, France

Carles Gaig MD
Parkinson's Disease and Movement
Disorders Unit, Neurology Service, Institut
Clínic de Neurociències, Hospital Clínic de
Barcelona, Universitat de Barcelona, Institut
d'Investigacions Biomèdiques August Pi I Sunyer
(IDIBAPS), Centro de Investigación Biomédica
en Red sobre Enfermedades Neurodegenerativas
(CIBERNED), Barcelona, Spain

Oscar S. Gershanik MD
Professor and Chairman, Department of
Neurology, Hospital Frances, Buenos Aires,
Argentina

Andreas Hartmann MD
Clinical Investigation Center, Pitié-Salpêtrière
Hospital; Federation of Nervous System Diseases,
Pitié-Salpêtrière Hospital; National Institute of
Health and Medical Research (INSERM U679);
Pierre et Marie Curie University, Paris, France

Robert A. Hauser MD
Professor of Neurology, Pharmacology and
Experimental Therapeutics; Director, Clinical
Neuroscience Research Program; Director,
Parkinson's Disease and Movement Disorders
Center of Excellence, University of South Florida,
Tampa, FL, USA

Alex Iranzo MD
Parkinson's Disease and Movement
Disorders Unit, Neurology Service, Institut
Clínic de Neurociències, Hospital Clínic de
Barcelona, Universitat de Barcelona, Institut
d'Investigacions Biomèdiques August Pi I Sunyer
(IDIBAPS), Centro de Investigación Biomédica
en Red sobre Enfermedades Neurodegenerativas
(CIBERNED), Barcelona, Spain

Georg H. Kägi MD
Sobell Department of Motor Neuroscience and
Movement Disorders, Institute of Neurology,
University College London, National Hospital
for Neurology and Neurosurgery, Queen Square,
London, UK

Christine Klein MD
Department of Neurology, University of Lübeck,
Lübeck, Germany

Anthony E. Lang MD
Director, Morton and Gloria Shulman Movement
Disorders Center, Toronto Western Hospital;
Director, Division of Neurology, University of
Toronto; Jack Clark Chair for Parkinson's Disease
Research, University of Toronto, Ontario, Canada

Matthias R. Lemke MD
Professor of Psychiatry, University of Kiel;
Department of Psychiatry, Kliniken Alsterdorf,
Hamburg, Germany

Irene Litvan MD
Raymond Lee Lebby Professor of Parkinson
Disease Research, Chief, Division of Movement
Disorders, University of Louisville School of
Medicine, Department of Neurology, Louisville,
KY, USA

Terry McClain MSN, ARNP
Parkinson's Disease and Movement Disorders
Center, University of South Florida, Tampa, FL,
USA

Wassilios Meissner MD, PhD
Department of Neurology, University Hospital
Haut-Lévêque, Bordeaux, France

Eldad Melamed MD
Department of Neurology, Rabin Medical
Center, Beilinson Campus, Petah Tiqwa, and
Sackler Faculty of Medicine, Tel Aviv University,
Tel Aviv, Israel

Wolfgang H. Oertel MD
Professor and Chairman, Department of
Neurology, Philipps-Universität, Marburg,
Germany

Werner Poewe MD
Professor and Chairman, Department of
Neurology, Medical University Innsbruck,
Austria

Pierre Pollak MD
Movement Disorders Unit, Pôle Neurologie-
Psychiatrie, University Hospital of Grenoble, and
Equipe Dynamique des Réseaux Neuronaux du
Mouvement Grenoble Institut des Neurosciences,
Grenoble, France

Anthony H.V. Schapira MD, DSc, FRCP, FMedSci
Head of Department, University Department of Clinical Neurosciences, Institute of Neurology, Queen Square, London; Professor of Neurology, National Hospital for Neurology and Neurosurgery, and Royal Free Hospital, London, UK

Frédéric Sedel MD, PhD
Federation of Nervous System Diseases, Hôpital de la Salpêtrière, Paris, France

Thomas D. L. Steeves MD
Division of Neurology, University of Toronto and the Morton and Gloria Shulman Movement Disorders Centre, Toronto Western Hospital, Toronto, Ontario, Canada

Matthew B. Stern MD
Parkinson's Disease and Movement Disorders Center, University of Pennsylvania; Philadelphia PADRECC (Parkinson's Disease Research Education & Clinical Center), Philadelphia, PA, USA

Fabrizio Stocchi MD, PhD
Department of Neurology, IRCCS San Raffaele, Rome, Italy

Heike Stockner MD
Department of Neurology, Medical University Innsbruck, Austria

Philip D. Thompson MB, PhD, FRACP
Discipline of Medicine, University of Adelaide, and Department of Neurology, Royal Adelaide Hospital, Adelaide, Australia

François Tison MD, PhD
Department of Neurology, University Hospital Haut-Lévêque, Bordeaux, France

Mathias Toft MD, PhD
Department of Neurology, Center of Clinical Neuroscience, Rikshospitalet University Hospital, Oslo, Norway

Eduardo Tolosa MD, FRCP
Parkinson's Disease and Movement Disorders Unit, Neurology Service, Institut Clínic de Neurociències, Hospital Clínic de Barcelona, Universitat de Barcelona, Institut d'Investigacions Biomèdiques August Pi I Sunyer (IDIBAPS), Centro de Investigación Biomédica en Red sobre Enfermedades Neurodegenerativas (CIBERNED), Barcelona, Spain

Jean-Marc Trocello MD
Centre de référence Bernard Pépin pour la maladie de Wilson, Department of Neurology, Lariboisière Hospital, Paris, France

André R. Troiano MD
Pierre et Marie Curie University; Federative Institute for Neuroscience Research; Department of Genetics and Cytogenetics, Pitié-Salpêtrière Hospital, Paris, France

Marcus M. Unger MD
Department of Neurology, Philipps-Universität, Marburg, Germany

Francesc Valldeoriola MD
Parkinson's Disease and Movement Disorders Unit, Neurology Service, Institut Clínic de Neurociències, Hospital Clínic de Barcelona, Universitat de Barcelona, Institut d'Investigacions Biomèdiques August Pi I Sunyer (IDIBAPS), Centro de Investigación Biomédica en Red sobre Enfermedades Neurodegenerativas (CIBERNED), Barcelona, Spain

Daniel Weintraub MD
Assistant Professor of Psychiatry and Neurology, University of Pennsylvania School of Medicine; Parkinson's Disease Research, Education and Clinical Center (PADRECC) and the Mental Illness Research, Education and Clinical Center (MIRECC), Philadelphia Veterans Affairs Medical Center, Philadelphia, PA, USA

Jayne R. Wilkinson MD
Parkinson's Disease and Movement Disorders Center, University of Pennsylvania; Philadelphia PADRECC (Parkinson's Disease Research Education & Clinical Center), Philadelphia, PA, USA

France Woimant MD
Centre de référence Bernard Pépin pour la
maladie de Wilson, Department of Neurology,
Lariboisière Hospital, Paris, France

Zbigniew K. Wszolek MD
Consultant and Professor of Neurology,
Department of Neurology, Mayo Clinic,
Jacksonville, FL, USA

Preface

Why, you may ask, yet another book on Parkinson's disease (PD) when excellent works for specialists and the general public already exist on the subject? Our answer is twofold. First, most are written as clinical neurology textbooks directed towards the practical management of the disease or from a neuroscientific perspective geared toward an understanding of disease fundamentals. Rarely, however, are the two approaches examined together. It was our view that both are essential components in disease management given that treatment of PD requires an excellent understanding of the brain's anatomy, physiology, and pharmacology. Secondly, with the many recent major discoveries in the field of basic and clinical research, an update of this information, particularly in the context of the novel and emerging therapies for PD, is timely.

What has become clear over the years is that PD is not a single anatomoclinical entity, but rather comprises a spectrum of several entities. Thus, it is now more appropriate to speak of Parkinson's *diseases*, and a collection of clinical features that may constitute a syndrome. Indeed, from now on, one must speak of parkinsonian syndrome given the multitude of clinical phenotypes, not to mention the many and varied histopathological features of the disorder that differ from one patient to another. That being the case, why use the name Parkinson for these diseases, a designation that has not changed since Jean-Martin Charcot first used it? At the time, it was a tribute to James Parkinson; later on, however, it became a habit as a result of grouping together all the clinical presentations under one illness. While far from perfect, it is probably still the best designation for a group of disorders that all have an akinetic-rigid syndrome.

Caring for PD patients implies first and foremost being sure of the diagnosis, offering as far as possible a prognosis, and then implementing treatment that can be adapted over time. This is a challenging task because the very notion of PD has changed much in recent decades. The history of PD can be schematically illustrated in four major successive stages. Since its initial description in 1817, PD has been considered a movement disorder, hence its place as the flagship disease of the Movement Disorder Society. In the 1970s and 1980s, the existence of cognitive disorders in PD was widely debated before being acknowledged. In the 1990s, the psychiatric aspects of the disorder came to the forefront. And today, we have finally come to understand that the disorder primarily impacts on quality of life and social integration, raising various public health issues.

The clinical presentation of PD, which can almost be described as a neuropsychiatric disorder, can be polymorphous, characterized by features that differ from one patient to another and vary over time. The neuropathological features are still not yet fully known and, as we shall see in the following chapters, include various brain lesions and histopathological stigmata not solely limited to Lewy bodies. Greater insight into the anatomicopharmacological mechanisms grows daily as evidence of both dopaminergic and non-dopaminergic lesions comes to light. The biochemical mechanisms involved in the neuronal dysfunction and death responsible for PD are countless and are not necessarily the primary causes of the disorder which may or may not be hereditary.

Hopefully, the reader can now appreciate why so many internationally renowned experts in the field were asked to contribute to what we believe is an original work. The book's intent is threefold. First, the book should be instructive: practitioners must be better able to treat patients on the basis of a rigorously defined semiological system and modern physiopathological interpretation thereof. Secondly, the book should also be practical: in other words, how during the consultation can a practitioner manage the patient in the best possible way? Lastly, the book should be interesting: hence the idea of presenting the reader with different clinical scenarios, both typical situations requiring a consensus or atypical ones involving extensive discussion.

This initiative, therefore, consists of three chapters. First, a compilation of the major brain lesions typically seen in PD. The second chapter seeks to summarize the treatment of PD, based upon the lessons learned in the first chapter. Then there are 25 case studies designed to test the reader and the practical application of the information supplied in the first two chapters. The aim is to summarize the main clinical symptoms, discuss other diagnostic possibilities, and cite the main anatomobiochemical defects in order to draw major treatment conclusions. The ultimate goal is that the reader should have an up-to-date, clear, and logical idea of what caring for parkinsonian patients entails – a challenge that will undoubtedly continue for many years to come.

Yves Agid, Anthony Schapira, Andreas Hartmann

Introduction

Contrary to what is often thought, *the management of parkinsonian patients is a complex, time-consuming, and difficult task.* First, because the therapeutic challenge includes not only the patient's physical and psychological well-being, but also the quality of life of the patient and his family and, perhaps even more importantly, his social integration within the family, the workplace, and society in general. Secondly, treatment is challenging because it must constantly be adapted as symptoms evolve with passing time. Whenever a physician sees a patient with probable or possible Parkinson's disease (PD), the same three nagging questions come to mind: Is the diagnosis correct? What does the future hold for the patient? Should symptomatic treatment be initiated or, if already in place, should it be modified? Patients and/or the persons who accompany them are almost always plagued by these questions, but very often they are too embarrassed or dare not ask them. The physician must, therefore, exercise tact to determine if these questions should be broached openly straight away or discussed more cautiously during subsequent consultations.

The diagnosis of PD is far from easy. Two different situations must be distinguished depending on whether the examination occurs early on in disease progression or later. At the onset of the disorder, there is a risk of confusing it with postural tremor, focal dystonia or an even rarer condition such as Wilson's disease. It is here that a precise semiological system is paramount in several ways. First, by listening to allow the patient to describe his main difficulties and his psychological pain. Next by adopting an overall, behavioral approach to the actual examination, namely by making the patient walk to observe his gait and then having him write ("the neurologist's two best tools are a smooth carpet and a pen"). Lastly, by being aware of certain examination maneuvers that can reveal resting tremor (mental counting) or rigidity (Froment's sign).

As PD progresses, most if not all patients are treated with levodopa or its derivatives. As a result, patients can suffer either from PD symptoms, from motor and psychiatric complications related to antiparkinsonian treatment, or often from both. Thus it is convenient to classify PD patients into three different categories: those who respond well to levodopa; those who do not; and those whose initial good response diminishes with time.

In approximately 15% of cases, patients experience dramatic improvement with levodopa. These forms of the disorder are sometimes characterized by severe motor complications combining various kinds of dyskinesia (monophasic, biphasic, "off"-period dystonia) and motor performance fluctuations (wearing-off, "on"/"off" periods), the very observation of which suggests the diagnosis of levodopa-responsive PD.

At the other extremity of the disorder spectrum are the 15% of patients who do not respond or respond only marginally to levodopa. These cases represent the "cousins" of classical PD within the framework of what is conventionally referred to as Parkinson-plus syndromes. Patients do not suffer from levodopa-related motor complications as the patients do not respond to replacement therapy. On the other hand, other typical symptoms are present, namely the so-called axial symptoms: dysexecutive syndrome or even dementia; ocular anomalies; dysarthria and swallowing problems; nuchal rigidity and postural problems; sphincter problems and dysautonomia; gait disorders and postural instability. While we can treat levodopa-responsive symptoms, there are few drugs that are effective against these other symptoms, hence the severity of Parkinson-plus syndromes.

In the remaining 70% of PD patients, symptoms respond well to replacement therapy initially. An apparent tolerance to treatment develops over time, however, as a result of non-dopaminergic lesions – obviously unresponsive to the restoration of dopaminergic transmission – that accumulate in the brain. One can understand, therefore, why it is essential for the neurologist to distinguish symptoms that respond to levodopa from those that do not. The former can be easily improved with various replacement therapies while the latter should benefit from other treatments (antidepressants, anxiolytics, physical and speech therapy, etc.).

Determining a prognosis on seeing a PD patient for the first time, especially early on in the disease, is even more difficult. Initially, there is the risk of misdiagnosis, although if the accepted criteria for PD are followed (asymmetric bradykinetic rigid syndrome with unilateral resting tremor that responds to levodopa treatment), the diagnosis is highly accurate. The observation of intellectual inertia, subtle memory deficits, axial rigidity, postural instability, urinary urge or incontinence and relative dopamine unresponsiveness indicates a rather poor prognosis. Most of the time, the response to replacement treatment with levodopa or dopamine derivatives must be waited for before reaching a decision (provided that the treatment is adequate and the patient adjusts to it well). In broad terms, although this is not always the case, young patients, particularly those with akinetic-rigid PD, respond dramatically to levodopa. They quickly develop motor complications (dyskinesias, "on"/"off" effects), however, that in some instances can be severe. Older patients tend to present with a slightly different form of PD, typically tremor-type PD, which, although not responding as well to replacement therapy with levodopa – a problem per se – presents fewer treatment-related motor complications. At this stage, namely once the adjustment to replacement therapy is at its best, it is primarily the evaluation of those symptoms that persist at the maximum effect of treatment that determine the prognosis. If the patient no longer has problems while on treatment, levodopa and its derivatives have a good chance of continued efficacy; if there is insufficient improvement of the motor impairment, primarily of the axial signs, the prognosis is probably poor. As for what the future holds for the patient and his family, extreme caution is de rigueur as one may be wrong. But it is also important for the patient that the positive aspects of treatment and the rapid pace of research in improving therapies be emphasized. The progression of motor, intellectual, and psychiatric disorders must be monitored during follow-up.

Treatment of parkinsonian symptoms implies a good knowledge of brain physiology. It is essential that the therapist have a solid understanding of basal ganglia neuronal dysfunction in PD, implying solid training in the fields of neuroanatomy, neurophysiology, and neuropharmacology. A very comprehensive therapeutic armamentarium is available to restore deficient dopaminergic transmission in the central nervous system. Levodopa, which is converted to dopamine, is the gold standard for treating PD. It is an effective and powerful drug, but not without side effects, primarily motor, that can be disabling. Other commonly used drugs are dopamine agonists which act directly at the dopamine receptor level and do not need to be converted to dopamine. Other adjuvant agents include catechol-*O*-methyltransferase inhibitors, monoamine oxidase B inhibitors, amantadine, and anticholinergics. By contrast, there is a dearth of drugs that improve symptoms unresponsive to or only marginally responsive to dopaminergic therapy, namely "axial" symptoms present at the outset in Parkinson-plus diseases or which can develop in some advanced forms of the disease. It is in such cases that psychotherapy and physical and speech therapy play an essential role.

Whatever the case, however, physicians recognize that commitment to treatment is for the patient's entire existence. Patient care implies discretion and judgment because every patient has specific, individual needs. It also demands a logical long-term strategy and strong personal involvement in order to ensure quality of life and social reintegration for both patients and their families.

1 What is Parkinson's disease? From pathophysiology to symptoms

Andreas Hartmann, Yves Agid, Anthony Schapira

What are the pathophysiological alterations underlying Parkinson's disease (PD) and how do these alterations translate into clinical symptoms? This is what this chapter aims to discuss. Specifically, we will define which dopaminergic and non-dopaminergic systems are affected in PD. Next, we will look at the consequences of this disease on brain circuitry. Then, we will ask why and how these pathophysiological alterations occur. Finally, we will examine the symptoms that result from these multiple cerebral dysfunctions. Understanding these links will enable the reader to make rational therapeutic decisions when treating PD patients based on how the brain dysfunctions.

I. Pathophysiology of Parkinson's disease

1. Dysfunctions of the main neuronal pathways in Parkinson's disease

Historically, PD has been considered a "motor" disease linked to degeneration of midbrain dopaminergic neurons. However, this assumption can no longer be maintained. PD is now known to be a disease with numerous non-motor symptoms that affects multiple, non-dopaminergic neuronal populations. "Non-motor" does not, however, equate with "non-dopaminergic." Motor symptoms are also provoked by dysfunctions of non-dopaminergic systems. With this in mind, the reader is prepared to enter the complexities of PD. Once these are understood, the therapeutic rationale in treating PD becomes apparent and logical.

a. An overview of neuronal systems affected in Parkinson's disease

Cellular loss in PD affects dopaminergic and non-dopaminergic neurons (Fig. 1.1). Dopaminergic neuronal loss can be subdivided into two categories: that affecting the nigrostriatal system where the brunt of the pathology occurs, and extra-nigrostriatal dopaminergic systems. The latter can be subdivided into three parts: (i) dopaminergic systems originating from the mesencephalon but targeting structures other than the dorsal striatum, i.e. the mesolimbic, mesocortical, and mesopallidal systems; (ii) dopaminergic neurons located

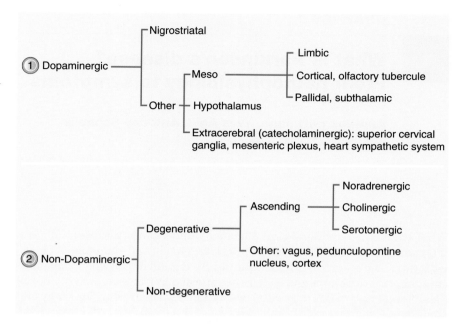

Figure 1.1 Overview of neuronal cell loss in Parkinson's disease.

outside the mesencephalon, e.g. the hypothalamus and parathalamic neurons projecting towards the spinal cord; and (iii) extracerebral dopaminergic neurons, e.g. the mesenteric plexus.

Non-dopaminergic neuronal loss is widespread and heterogeneous. It can be subdivided into degenerative lesions of (i) ascending noradrenergic, serotonergic, and cholinergic ascending neuronal systems, and (ii) of the nucleus vagus, the peduncolopontine nucleus, and neurons of the cerebral cortex. Finally, additional non-degenerative lesions, independent of the primary pathological process, such as diffuse white matter lesions sometimes seen in aged patients, may also contribute to the clinical picture in PD.

b. Dopaminergic neurons

Dopaminergic neurons can be found in multiple areas of the central nervous system. To understand the symptoms of PD, it is helpful to separate mesencephalic from extra-mesencephalic dopaminergic populations.

In PD patients, the loss of dopaminergic neurons in the midbrain is *selective*. The characteristic pathological changes are the loss of pigmented dopaminergic neurons, particularly in the ventral tier of the substantia nigra pars compacta (80–90%), less so in the ventral tegmental area (40–50%), and minimal (2–3%) in the central gray substance (Fig. 1.2). The loss of dopaminergic neurons in the substantia nigra pars compacta is responsible for the dopamine deficiency in the dorsal and anterior striatum, the putamen being more af-

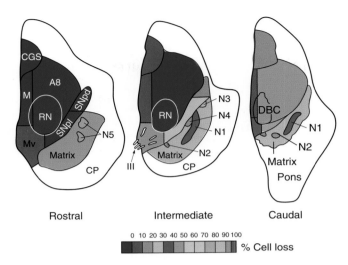

Rostral   Intermediate   Caudal

0 10 20 30 40 50 60 70 80 90 100
% Cell loss

Figure 1.2 Regional and intranigral loss of dopamine-containing neurons in Parkinson's disease. Cell loss: CGS (2–3%); Mv (40–50%); SN 80–90%. A8, dopaminergic cell group A8; CGS, central gray substance; CP, cerebral peduncle; DBC, decussation of brachium conjunctivum; M, medial group; Mv, medioventral group; N, nigrosome; RN, red nucleus; SNpd, substantia nigra pars dorsalis; SNpl, substantia nigra pars lateralis; III, exiting fibers of the third cranial nerve. The colorimetric scale indicates the estimated amount of cell loss (least = blue; most = red). Across the mesencephalon, dopaminergic cell loss was weak in the central gray substance and the red nucleus, and intermediate in the dopaminergic cell group A8 and the medioventral group of the ventral tegmental area. Within the substantia nigra pars compacta, dopamine-containing neurons in the calbindin-rich regions ("matrix") and in five calbindin-poor pockets ("nigrosomes") were identified. The spatiotemporal progression of neuronal loss in the substantia nigra pars compacta is as follows: depletion begins in the main pocket (nigrosome 1) and then spreads to other nigrosomes and the matrix along rostral, medial and dorsal axes of progression. Adapted from Damier P, Hirsch EC, Agid Y, Graybiel AM. *Brain* 1999; 122(Pt8): 1437–48.

fected than the caudate nucleus. It is the nigrostriatal dopaminergic pathway that contributes to the control of motor functions and its disruption results in the classic PD motor triad (akinesia/bradykinesia, rigidity, and rest tremor).

Although it is generally assumed that at least 50% of dopaminergic neurons in the substantia nigra pars compacta must degenerate before symptoms appear, this is an oversimplification. In fact, nigral dopaminergic neurons degenerate heterogeneously in the substantia nigra with some areas heavily burdened by pathology and others that remain functional until late in the disease course (Fig. 1.3). For symptoms to occur, specific areas within the substantia nigra may lose up to 90% of dopaminergic neurons with an accordingly drastic reduction in striatal dopamine concentrations at precise somatotopic locations (Fig. 1.4). This explains why PD symptoms manifest in restricted parts of the body (mainly the distal limbs) at the beginning of the disease and then extend bilaterally to the remaining parts of the body.

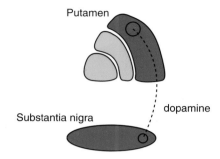

Figure 1.3 Selective symptoms in Parkinson's disease originate from discrete cell loss. Dopaminergic neurons in the substantia nigra degenerate in regions linked to specific areas in the putamen that cause selective symptoms in Parkinson's disease.

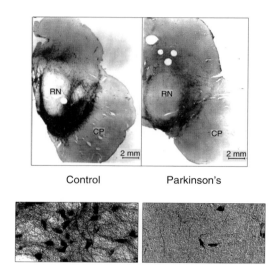

Figure 1.4 Depletion of dopaminergic neurons in the substantia nigra in Parkinson's disease. Upper panel, tyrosine hydroxylase (TH) staining (as an indicator of dopamine content) of the mesencephalon. In control subjects, TH staining is strong and confluent in the substantia nigra, whereas it is much weaker and spotted in Parkinson's disease patients. Microscopically, this is reflected by a much lower density of dopaminergic neurons (lower panel). Also note that dopaminergic neurons in Parkinson's disease are shrunken, and that significantly fewer dopaminergic fibers can be detected. Images courtesy of Etienne Hirsch, INSERM UMR 679, Hôpital de la Pitié-Salpêtrière, Paris, France.

Besides the degeneration of the nigrostriatal dopaminergic pathway, other dopaminergic neuronal pathways degenerate in the disease: the mesolimbic pathway projecting to limbic brain areas, especially the ventral striatum and the nucleus accumbens; the mesocortical pathway innervating the cerebral cortex; and the mesopallidal pathway connecting the substantia nigra to the pallidum (Fig. 1.5). Neuronal loss within these dopaminergic pathways is less

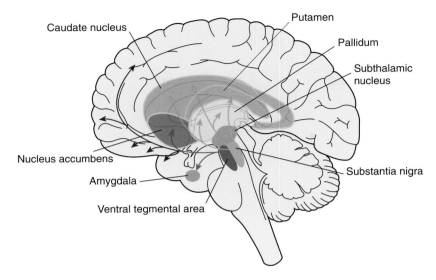

Figure 1.5 Dopaminergic pathways. Dopamine is the principal neurotransmitter in three major neuronal systems in the midbrain: the nigrostriatal pathway (orange), the mesolimbic system (red) and the mesocortical pathway (blue).

severe and variable across subjects, and contributes to mood (mesolimbic), cognitive (mesocortical), and motor (mesopallidal) disturbances.

Dopaminergic systems outside the mesencephalon are also affected in PD, albeit to a lesser degree, such as parathalamic neurons projecting to the spinal cord (potentially involved in restless legs syndrome) and hypothalamic neurons resulting in endocrine disturbances.

Catecholaminergic neurons outside the central nervous system may also degenerate, in particular dopaminergic neurons in the gut (plexus mesentericus) and noradrenergic nerve terminals in the heart (resulting in cardiac sympathetic denervation). These pathological alterations are assumed to play a role in dysautonomic symptoms such as neurogenic orthostatic hypotension and gastrointestinal motility disorders.

c. Non-dopaminergic neurons
Widespread and progressive neurodegeneration in the PD brain affects non-dopaminergic neurons, leading to the emergence of a variety of both motor and non-motor features. Ascending neuronal pathways originating from the raphe nucleus, the locus coeruleus, and the nucleus basalis of Meynert degenerate in PD (Fig. 1.6). As a result of these lesions, the serotonergic, noradrenergic, and cholinergic ascending neuronal systems are damaged. Symptoms include depression, apathy, and cognitive impairment. Other neurons are lost in the brainstem (nucleus vagus, pedunculopontine nucleus) and in the cerebral cortex. Their respective contribution to parkinsonian symptomatology

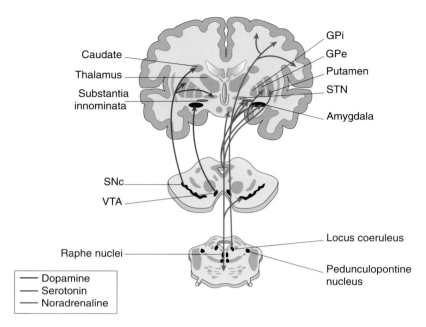

Caudate
Thalamus
Substantia
innominata

GPi
GPe
Putamen
STN
Amygdala

SNc
VTA

Raphe nuclei

Locus coeruleus
Pedunculopontine
nucleus

—— Dopamine
—— Serotonin
—— Noradrenaline

Figure 1.6 Multicentric neurodegeneration in Parkinson's disease. STN, subthalamic nucleus; GPi, globus pallidus internal segment; GPe, external segment; SNc, substantia nigra *pars compacta*; VTA, ventral tegmental area. The figure is a schematic representation of the monoamine neurotransmitter pathways (except for acetylcholine) affected in Parkinson's disease. "Non-dopaminergic" clinical manifestations in PD are probably caused by the loss of neurons in many cortical, subcortical, brainstem, and peripheral autonomic sites owing to the same neurodegenerative process that affects the nigrostriatal system. Reprinted from *The Lancet Neurology*, Vol. 3, Lang AE, Obeso JA. Current challenges in Parkinson's disease: restoring the nigrostriatal dopamine system will not suffice, pp. 309–16. Copyright 2004, with permission from Elsevier.

includes baroreflex failure, gait and posture abnormalities, and cortical dementia.

Non-degenerative lesions such as diffuse white matter abnormalities, considered to be of vascular origin, may also contribute to the clinical picture of PD. These lesions are non-specific, but they must be taken into account with regard to treatment response and prognosis (see below).

Further reading

Fearnley JM, Lees AJ. Ageing and Parkinson's disease: substantia nigra regional selectivity. *Brain* 1991; **114**(Pt 5): 2283–301.

Damier P, Hirsch EC, Agid Y, Graybiel AM. The substantia nigra of the human brain. II. Patterns of loss of dopamine-containing neurons in Parkinson's disease. *Brain* 1999; **122**(Pt 8): 1437–48.

Lang AE, Obeso JA. Time to move beyond nigrostriatal dopamine deficiency in Parkinson's disease. *Ann Neurol* 2004; **55**(6): 761–5.

2. Consequences of dopaminergic neuronal lesions on basal ganglia circuits

a. The dopaminergic nigrostriatal system: pre- and postsynaptic compensatory mechanisms

PD symptoms appear only after considerable degeneration of the dopaminergic nigrostriatal system, i.e. a 50% neuronal loss in the substantia nigra and 80% depletion of striatal dopamine. This means that there is a substantial presymptomatic period of the disease, during which major compensatory mechanisms take place delaying the appearance of symptoms. To date, these mechanisms have been studied exclusively in the nigrostriatal system and with the help of animal models of PD. It is plausible, however, to assume that similar mechanisms may also play a role in other dopaminergic and non-dopaminergic systems affected in PD.

These compensatory mechanisms can be subdivided into two sorts: pre- and postsynaptic. Presynaptically, compensation for dopaminergic cell loss in the substantia nigra may occur at the level of the cell body, the axon, and the synapse. Specifically, it has been proposed that (i) increased dopamine synthesis and turnover in the remaining nigral dopaminergic neurons, (ii) sprouting of dopaminergic (and possibly serotonergic) fibers in the striatum (axogenesis), and (iii) increased synaptic contacts (synaptogenesis) may occur. All three processes may be regulated by retrograde transport of trophic factors originating from striatal GABAergic neurons and/or surrounding astrocytes. Postsynaptically, striatal D_1 and D_2 receptor up-regulation may contribute to compensation of early nigral dopaminergic cell loss. In later disease stages, these same modifications of receptor sensitivity, especially D_1 (see below), may contribute to the emergence of motor fluctuations.

Research into the respective contribution of these mechanisms is ongoing. It is probable that these are active beyond the presymptomatic disease phase and, perhaps more importantly, may form the basis for new therapeutic strategies in PD.

Further reading

Mounayar S, Boulet S, Tande D *et al.* A new model to study compensatory mechanisms in MPTP-treated monkeys exhibiting recovery. *Brain* 2007; **130**(Pt 11): 2898–914.

Agid Y, Javoy-Agid F, Ruberg M. Biochemistry of neurotransmitters in Parkinson's disease. In: Marsden CD, Fahn S, eds. *Movement Disorders 2*. London: Butterworth, 1987:166–230.

b. Pathologic alterations of nigrostriatal circuits in Parkinson's disease

The consequences of dopaminergic lesions (*lesion* being defined as cell loss, rather than histopathological features such as inclusion bodies, see below), specifically those affecting the nigrostriatal pathway, have come under intense research over the past two decades. Importantly, they have made it possible to identify targets for functional neurosurgery in PD. In contrast, the brain circuit dysfunctions resulting from non-dopaminergic lesions remain widely unexplored, possibly because the contribution of these lesions to parkinsonian symptomatology has only recently aroused renewed interest. Thus, the following section will focus on basal ganglia circuits affected by dysfunctions of the nigrostriatal system.

Nigral dopaminergic neurons are linked to striatal neurons by postsynaptic dopamine receptors. These are characterized by ligand specificity and coupling to adenylate cyclase, and are subdivided into two classes: D1 and D2. The D1 class stimulates the adenylate cyclase pathway while the D2 class inhibits it. These neurons can also be distinguished by their specific neuropeptide content, i.e. dynorphin and substance P for D1 receptors, and enkephalin for D2 receptors. Currently, five human dopamine receptors have been identified: subtypes D_1 and D_5 in the D1 family, and subtypes D_2, D_3, and D_4 in the D2 family. D_1 and D_2 receptor activation produces synergistic effects in the striatum. The antiparkinsonian effects of most dopamine agonists are related to the stimulation of D_2 receptors, whereas mixed D_1/D_2 agonist activity may be important for a full reversal of PD motor deficits. This is why the effects of levodopa on motor function are usually superior to those of dopamine agonists. It is also believed, however, that stimulation of D_1 receptors partly underlies the occurrence of dyskinesia, explaining why most dopamine agonists are less likely to cause these motor complications than levodopa (Chapter 3, case study 11).

D_3 and D_4 receptors are more selectively associated with limbic brain areas, mainly associated with emotional functions, which receive their dopamine input from the ventral tegmental area (Chapter 3, case study 12). D_5 receptors are expressed in the hippocampus, the hypothalamus and the parafascicular nucleus of the thalamus, with as yet unclear functional consequences in PD.

When striatal dopaminergic deafferentiation of D_1 and D_2 receptors occurs, the basal ganglia circuitry is profoundly altered. The basal ganglia consist of the caudate nucleus, the putamen, the globus pallidus (subdivided into an internal and external part), and the subthalamic nucleus. The caudate and putamen together are called the striatum, which is the target of cortical input to the basal ganglia. The globus pallidus is the source of output to the thalamus. The basic motor circuit of the basal ganglia is a loop where information cycles from the cerebral cortex through the basal ganglia and thalamus, and then back to the cortex, particularly the supplementary motor area. One of the main functions of this loop seems to be the selection and automatic execution of voluntary movement. In addition, there are associative and limbic territories within the basal ganglia organized in loops which mainly control cognitive and emotional functions.

Figure 1.7 represents the classic model of the basal ganglia motor circuit in normal and parkinsonian states. This model proposes that the striatum, the major input region of the basal ganglia, is connected to the major output region, the globus pallidus (internal part) and the substantia nigra (pars reticulata), by a "direct" pathway (considered to be D_1 receptor-dependent) and by an "indirect" pathway (considered to be D_2 receptor-dependent) that has synaptic connections with the globus pallidus (external part) and the subthalamic nucleus (Chapter 3, case study 13). In normal subjects (Fig. 1.7a), dopaminergic neurons in the substantia nigra act to excite inhibitory neurons in the direct

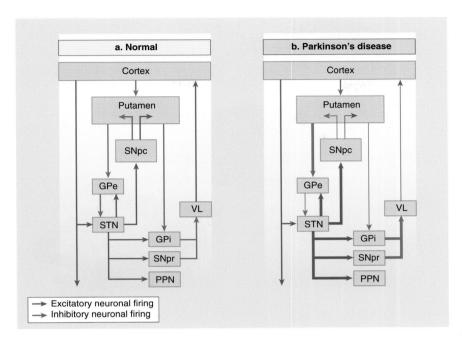

Figure 1.7 Basal ganglia circuit: classic model in normal subjects (a) and in Parkinson's disease (b). In parkinsonism, dopaminergic cell loss in the substantia nigra *pars compacta* (SNpc) globally results in a disinhibition of basal ganglia output structures, notably the subthalamic nucleus (STN) and globus pallidus internal (GPi), which are the prime targets for functional neurosurgery in PD. GPe, external global pallidus; SNpr, substantia nigra pars reticulata; PPN, pendunculopontine nucleus; VL, ventral lateral nucleus.

pathway and inhibit the excitatory influence of the indirect pathway. In PD (Fig. 1.7b), dopamine depletion leads to overactivity in the globus pallidus (internal part) and substantia nigra (pars reticulata) with excess inhibition of the thalamus and reduced activation of cortical motor regions, which translate into the development of parkinsonian features.

Although this model has many merits, the past decade has also shown that it contains errors and unanswered questions. For example, while hypoactivity of the direct pathway has been confirmed experimentally, hyperactivity of the indirect pathway remains a subject of debate. Moreover, recent studies call into question the exclusive segregation of the direct and indirect pathways. They report a larger amount of collateralization between both pathways in primates than that reported for rodent basal ganglia. Furthermore, recent studies suggest that motor, associative, and limbic territories within the basal ganglia territories are separated by functional gradients, not by sharp boundaries, and converge from the cortex to the striatum to the globus pallidus and finally the subthalamic nucleus. The subthalamic nucleus may, therefore, represent a nexus for the integration of motor, cognitive and emotional aspects of

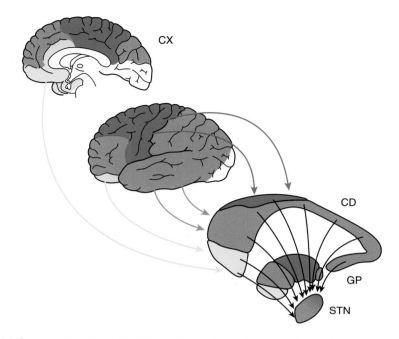

Figure 1.8 Schematic illustration of the convergence of projections from the cerebral cortex (CX), caudate nucleus (CD), and globus pallidus (GP) on the subthalamic nucleus (STN). These projections can be divided into three functional territories – sensorimotor (green), associative (mauve), and limbic (yellow) – and converge in the STN. Adapted from Mallet L, Schüpbach M, N'Diaye K, *et al. Proc Natl Acad Sci USA* 2007; **104**(25):10661–6.

behavior (Fig. 1.8). This explains the primary role of the subthalamic nucleus as the target for deep brain stimulation in basal ganglia disorders other than PD, such as obsessive-compulsive disorder. Conversely, the integrative functions of the subthalamic nucleus may also underlie psychiatric disturbances following deep brain stimulation.

Further reading

Graybiel AM. The basal ganglia: learning new tricks and loving it. *Curr Opin Neurobiol* 2005; **15**(6): 638–44.

Levesque M, Parent A. The striatofugal fiber system in primates: a reevaluation of its organization based on single-axon tracing studies. *Proc Natl Acad Sci USA* 2005; **102**(33): 11888–93.

3. Histopathology of Parkinson's disease

The histopathological criteria for PD are given in Table 1.1. In contrast to progressive supranuclear palsy, a Parkinson-plus syndrome, there are no tau-positive inclusions in PD. Senile plaques, as seen in Alzheimer's disease, can be observed in PD brains, especially in cortical areas. Gliosis, as a conse-

Table 1.1 Proposed criteria for histopathological confirmation of Parkinson's disease

---

1   Substantial nerve cell loss with accompanying gliosis in the substantia nigra.
2   At least one Lewy body in the substantia nigra or in the locus coeruleus. (Note: it may be necessary to examine up to four non-overlapping sections in each of these areas before concluding that Lewy bodies are absent.)
3   No pathological evidence for other diseases that produce parkinsonism, e.g. progressive supranuclear palsy, multiple system atrophy, corticobasal degeneration. (Note: in excluding other diseases that produce parkinsonism, published consensus criteria should be used when available.)

---

http://www.medicalcriteria.com/criteria/neuro_parkinson.htm

quence of cell death, occurs in several brain regions in PD, particularly in the substantia nigra. It is the presence of nigral and cortical Lewy bodies (Fig. 1.9), however, that plays a paramount role in diagnosing PD. Yet, they are not pathognomic for PD and can be observed in other parkinsonian syndromes such as multiple system atrophy or dementia with Lewy bodies. Lewy bodies are cytoplasmic inclusions consisting of a large variety of proteins such as α-synuclein (the main constituent), synphilin-1, ubiquitin, neurofilaments, oxidized/nitrated proteins, parkin, proteasomal elements, and heat shock proteins, among others.

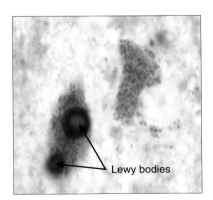
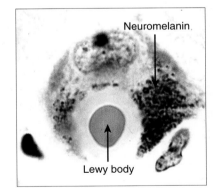

Figure 1.9 Lewy bodies in Parkinson's disease. The characteristic histopathological changes in PD are the loss of pigmented dopaminergic neurons, particularly in the ventral tier of the substantia nigra pars compacta, and the presence of Lewy bodies in a proportion of the surviving neurons. Lewy bodies are intracytoplasmic inclusions measuring 5–30 μm in diameter. They often have a dense hyaline eosinophilic core composed of concentric lamellae, surrounded by a pale halo. The Lewy body is composed of a number of different proteins that exhibit staining for ubiquitin, α-synuclein and proteasomal components. If on close examination of several sections of the midbrain, no Lewy bodies are found in the substantia nigra, a diagnosis of PD can usually be excluded and other causes of parkinsonism considered. Images courtesy of JJ Hauw, Department of Neuropathology, Hôpital de la Pitié-Salpêtrière, Paris, France.

In recent years, the staging of Lewy body distribution (by detection of intracellular α-synuclein-positive inclusion bodies) across the brain in PD by Braak and colleagues has received widespread attention (Table 1.2). This staging provides an elegant explanation for the occurrence both of motor and non-motor symptoms in PD, and maybe more importantly for the *kinetics* of symptom appearance.

Table 1.2 Progression of neurodegeneration in Parkinson's disease according to Braak and coworkers

Braak stage		Lesion sites	Clinical features
1		• Mostly, medulla oblongata ◦ Dorsal IX/X motor nucleus ◦ and/or intermediate reticular zone • Frequently, anterior olfactory nucleus	• The areas involved in the preclinical stage 1 and 2 are thought to be key areas that mediate non-motor symptoms such as ◦ olfactory dysfunction (hyposmia) ◦ sleep disturbances (RBD*; restless legs syndrome) ◦ other autonomic abnormalities
2		• Caudal raphe nuclei • Gigantocellular reticular nucleus • Coeruleus-subcoeruleus complex	
3		• Midbrain ◦ Substantia nigra pars compacta ◦ Other deep nuclei of the midbrain	• Typical PD triad ◦ Tremor ◦ Rigidity ◦ Bradykinasia

4		• Forebrain
		 ◦ Basal prosencephalon
		 ◦ Mesocortex
		  − Temporal mesocortex
		  − Allocortex
		(neocortex is unaffected)	

5		• Neocortex ◦ High order sensory association areas of neocortex ◦ Prefrontal neocortex	• Neuropsychiatric symptoms • Cognitive impairment
6		• Neocortex ◦ First order sensory association areas ◦ Premotor areas ◦ Primary sensory areas (occasionally) ◦ Primary motor field (occasionally)	

* RBD, rapid eye movement (REM) behavioral disorder

The traditional view that the pathological process in PD initiates with the degeneration of dopaminergic neurons in the substantia nigra is challenged by Braak and colleagues who introduced the concept of a six-stage neuropathological process allowing differentiation of initial, intermediate, and final stages of PD-related histopathological lesions. The table displays this staging, which is based on distribution of α-synuclein-positive inclusion bodies (not neuronal degeneration) throughout the brain. Based on Braak H, Rüb U, Gai WP, Del Tredici K. *J Neural Transm* 2003; **110**: 517–36.

Braak stage 1 denotes Lewy body deposition of the olfactory bulb and the anterior olfactory nucleus, which can clinically manifest as olfactory dysfunction. Braak stage 2 characterizes progression of the pathological process to the lower brainstem. These areas, implicated in the preclinical stages 1 and 2 of PD, are also thought to be key areas that mediate non-motor symptoms such as olfaction, sleep homoeostasis, and autonomic symptoms. For instance, sleep might be affected by abnormalities in the sleep–wake cycle-related pathway that mediates thalamocortical arousal, including brainstem nuclei such as the raphe nucleus (serotonin) and the locus coeruleus (noradrenaline). The locus coeruleus, subcoeruleus nucleus, and raphe nucleus are also thought to be key areas related to the origin of visual hallucinations and rapid eye movement (REM) sleep behavior disorder in PD (Chapter 3, case studies 1 and 6). Furthermore, medullary nuclei, which play an important part in central autonomic control, may be affected at this stage, explaining early autonomic disturbances in PD.

The typical motor triad of akinesia, rigidity, and rest tremor only emerge at Braak stages 3 and 4 when the neurodegenerative process has affected the substantia nigra. This stage is when "true" neurodegeneration (as evidenced by cell loss rather than the presence of Lewy bodies) first occurs in PD and crosses the threshold from a premotor to a motor disorder. The final two stages, Braak stages 5 and 6, correlate with the presence of Lewy bodies in limbic structures and the neocortex. Patients may have neuropsychiatric symptoms such as depression, cognitive impairment, and visual hallucinations at this stage.

However, justified criticisms of this model have been raised. Specifically, the presence of Lewy bodies is not necessarily a sign of neuronal damage, and "genuine" lesions involving neuronal loss in extranigral areas have been described in PD, but their chronological appearance remains unknown. In line with this, one of the central questions in PD pathophysiology remains whether Lewy bodies cause cell death, prevent cell death, or are mere bystanders. A recent and intriguing hypothesis suggests that accelerated formation of nonfibrillar α-synuclein oligomers is the critical process in PD pathogenesis. These oligomers are precursors of Lewy bodies, suggesting that Lewy body formation may even be *neuroprotective* by sequestering the toxic species. Alternatively, Lewy bodies may occur as an *epiphenomenon* of the primary pathology and have little or no effect on neuronal viability. Finally, Lewy bodies may be *toxic,* since they are composed of abnormal neurofilaments and their presence may indicate a general aberration of the cytoskeleton. In addition, entrapment of vital cellular organelles and inhibition of axonal transport by Lewy bodies have been described.

While awaiting answers to these questions, the Braak staging remains a hypothetical model of neuronal dysfunction related to the presence of α-synuclein-positive neuronal inclusions. For now, it is safe to assume that the presence of Lewy bodies can be considered a "fingerprint" of past or present neuronal suffering, and thus remains a valid hallmark of PD.

Further reading
Braak H, Bohl JR, Muller CM, Rub U, de Vos RA, Del Tredici K. Stanley Fahn Lecture 2005: The staging procedure for the inclusion body pathology associated with sporadic Parkinson's disease reconsidered. *Mov Disord* 2006; **21**(12): 2042–51.
Halliday GM, McCann H. Human-based studies on alpha-synuclein deposition and relationship to Parkinson's disease symptoms. *Exp Neurol* 2008; **209**(1): 12–21.
Harrower TP, Michell AW, Barker RA. Lewy bodies in Parkinson's disease: protectors or perpetrators? *Exp Neurol* 2005; **195**(1): 1–6.

4. The etiopathogenesis of Parkinson's disease

The development of successful disease-modifying therapies depends upon an exact understanding of the pathogenesis of PD. Effective "neuroprotective" therapies will hopefully delay or prevent degeneration of dopaminergic *and* non-dopaminergic pathways. Multiple cellular alterations leading to neuronal demise have been identified to date. Schematically, two main pathways of cell toxicity coexist. The first pathway is related to protein misfolding and aggregation, either as a consequence of an increased production (e.g. α-synuclein aggregation) or decreased elimination (proteasomal dysfunction) of toxic proteins. The second pathway is related to mitochondrial dysfunction, especially of the mitochondrial respiratory chain. Both pathways ultimately lead to an increase in oxidative stress and intracellular energy depletion (Fig. 1.10).

Another important notion relates to the selective vulnerability of neurons to undergo cell death, especially dopaminergic neurons. In particular, dopamine metabolism, neuromelanin accumulation, iron content, and decreased concentrations in anti-oxidant enzymes, all resulting in free radical formation, are obvious vulnerability factors for the degeneration of dopaminergic neurons. In recent years, the glial microenvironment has also been increasingly recognized as a potential vulnerability factor for nigral dopaminergic neurons.

All these alterations and vulnerability factors are believed to be caused either by genetic and/or environmental factors. Their consequence in terms of cell death are probably equal; not so the therapeutic consequences, which are more complex.

a. The genetics of Parkinson's disease: any clues for the sporadic forms?

Until the late 1990s, PD was considered to be a sporadic disease. In a significant number of cases (10–15%), however, the disease runs in families without a clear-cut Mendelian pattern of inheritance. This observation suggests that in such patients, PD is a complex trait determined by several genetic as well as non-genetic factors. More rarely, the PD phenotype is transmitted as a Mendelian trait, with either autosomal dominant or recessive inheritance (Table 1.3). Of note, non-genetic factors and disease modifiers that modulate the penetration of a certain mutation, onset age, and clinical features may still be critical in these patients (Chapter 3, case studies 22 and 24).

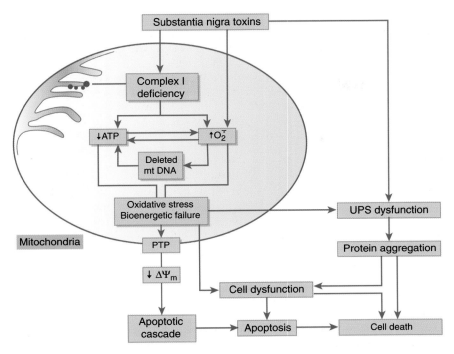

Figure 1.10 Mitochondrial dysfunction and cell death. ATP, adenosine triphosphate; PTP, permeability transition pore; UPS, ubiquitin proteasome system; $\Delta\Psi m$, Mitochondrial membrane potential.

In light of these findings, our view on PD has changed in three major aspects.

First, it is hoped that understanding the function of the proteins encoded by mutated genes may deepen our understanding of pathophysiological alterations relevant to the *sporadic* disease form. Alpha-synuclein is an illustration of that principle, as this gene is both mutated in autosomal-dominantly inherited forms of PD, and the encoded protein is also the main constituent of Lewy bodies in sporadic PD. In a similar vein, genes responsible for early-onset autosomal-recessive parkinsonism have pointed towards major intracellular mechanisms involved in nigral dopaminergic neurodegeneration: Parkin as a ubiquitin ligase points to the importance of the proteasome degradation machinery; PTEN-induced putative kinase 1 (*PINK1*) as a mitochondrial protein kinase points to the importance of mitochondrial dysfunction; *DJ1* as a sensor for oxidative stress points to the deleterious actions of reactive oxygen species for nigral cellular survival.

Second, although many genetic forms are exceedingly rare, some are sufficiently common to be relevant in everyday clinical practice. For example, the

Table 1.3 Genes identified in familial forms of Parkinson's disease with Mendelian inheritance

Locus	Chromosomal region	Gene	Putative biological significance of the abnormal protein	Age of onset	Inheritance	Clinical phenotype
PARK1	4q21-q23	α-synuclein	α-synuclein is one of the principal components of Lewy bodies. Mutant isoforms of alpha synuclein aggregate more readily. It has been suggested that their tendency to aggregate into misfolded structures may confer toxic properties to the protein	Young	AD	Similar to idiopathic PD (IPD), rapid progression
PARK2	6q25.2-q27	Parkin	Parkin functions as an E3 ligase, ubiquitinating proteins for destruction by the proteasome; accumulation of ubiquitinated, insoluble and unfolded forms of a normal substrate	Young	AR	Symptomatic improvement following sleep, mild dystonia, good response to levodopa, slow progression
PARK3	2p13	Unknown	–	Similar to IPD	AD	Dopa-responsive parkinsonism with a mean age at onset of 59 years
PARK4	4p15.1	Unknown	–	Young	AD	Rapidly progressive, dopa-responsive parkinsonism in early or mid-30s; early-stage weight loss, dementia in later stages
PARK5	4p14	UCHL1	Impaired protein clearance through ubiquitin–proteasome systems	Similar to IPD	AD	Similar to IPD

PARK6	1p35-p36	PINK1	Altered phosphorylation of target mitochondrial proteins leading to abnormal stress response and neurodegeneration	Young	AR	Benign course, levodopa-responsive
PARK7	1p36	DJ1	Impairment of protection against toxicity mediated by free radicals	Young	AR	Levodopa-responsive
PARK8	12q12	LRRK2	Dysregulation of cytoskeletal responses to external stimuli and vesicular trafficking	Similar to IPD	AD	Similar to IPD (LRRK2 mutations are the commonest cause of either familial or "sporadic" PD)
PARK9	1p36	ATP13A2	–	Young	AR	Levodopa-responsive parkinsonism with additional features such as spasticity, dementia, or supranuclear gaze paralysis
PARK10	1p32	Unknown	–	25–75 years	?	Similar to IPD
PARK11	2q36-q37	Unknown	–	60	?	Unknown
PARK12	Xq21-q25	Unknown	-	Similar to IPD	X-linked	Unknown
PARK13	2p12	Omi/HtrA2	Serine protease targeted to mitochondria	Similar to IPD	AD	Levodopa-responsive parkinsonism

Abbreviations: AD, autosomal dominant; AR, autosomal recessive; UCH-L1, ubiquitin carboxy-terminal hydrolase L1; PINK1, phosphatase and tensin homolog deleted on chromosome 10 (PTEN)-induced kinase 1; LRRK2, leucine-rich repeat kinase 2; IPD, idiopathic Parkinson's disease.

autosomal-dominant leucine-rich repeat kinase 2 (*LRRK2*) mutations account for 1–2% of sporadic cases in most European populations, with even higher figures in North African Arabs, Ashkenazi Jews, and Chinese populations. Importantly, *LRRK2* cases may be clinically undistinguishable from idiopathic PD and owing to incomplete penetrance, a clear family history is not always apparent. If these results are confirmed in subsequent series, *LRRK2* mutations will become the first genetic test with relevance for patients with the typical, late-onset form of PD.

Third, genes mutated in monogenic variants of PD may also play a role in a large proportion of patients without clear Mendelian inheritance. These genetic effects are mediated by common variants (polymorphisms) that cause subtle alterations in gene expression and/or the function of the encoded protein. These polymorphisms are not disease-causing mutations in the classic sense, but may predispose an individual to develop PD, either in combination with other gene polymorphisms or with external, environmental causes ("multiple hit" hypothesis of PD). Furthermore, genes not implicated in familial PD forms may play a role as susceptibility factors. One recent example is the glucocerebrosidase gene which is mutated in Gaucher's disease but may cause or at least predispose to PD in certain populations, i.e. Ashkenazi Jews (Table 1.4) (Chapter 3, case study 19).

The importance of genetic testing is therefore expected to increase in the near future for patients presenting with parkinsonism. Despite the importance of genetic studies for the research into the etiopathogenesis of PD, however, their utility in clinical practice for diagnostic or predictive (presymptomatic) purposes remains a matter of debate. As long as specific treatments are not available for PD patients carrying a certain gene mutation, genetic testing bears no immediate practical consequences for the management of these patients.

Table 1.4 Other genes associated with PD and parkinsonism

N-acetyltransferase 2 (*NAT2*)
Nuclear receptor related 1 (*NURR1*)
Cytochrome P450 2D6 (*CYP2D6*)
Dopamine D2 receptor gene (*DRD2*)
Monoamine oxidase B (*MAOB*)
Ferritin (light chain)
Glutathione S-transferase theta 1 (*GSTT1*)
Tau H1 haplotype
Glucocerebrosidase beta (*GBA*)
Synuclein alpha (SNCA) (*PARK1*) promoter polymorphism
UCHL1 (*PARK5*) polymorphism
Spinocerebellar ataxia (*SCA3*)

Mutations of these genes may not be causative, but rather predispose an individual to develop PD, possibly in association with other genes and/or environmental factors.

b. Relevant environmental factors: focus on mitochondria

Support for an environmental etiology of PD comes from the occurrence of post-encephalitic parkinsonism, from two known geographical clusters of PD-like neurodegenerative diseases (the "Guam complex" and "Guadeloupean parkinsonism"), and from the discovery of toxic models of parkinsonism caused by 1-methyl-4-phenyl-1,2,3,6-tetrahydropyridine (MPTP) and rotenone. Furthermore, there is possibly an epidemiological association of common PD with environmental factors such as rural living and occupational exposure to pesticides. Finally, as discussed above, genetic susceptibility factors may interact with environmental toxins ("multiple hit" hypothesis of PD).

Many pesticides, as well as MPTP, rotenone, and annonacin (the causative agent in Guadeloupean parkinsonism) are inhibitors of complex I in the mitochondrial respiratory chain. Complex I deficiency has long been recognized in sporadic PD, although its cause remains unknown in the absence of clear toxin exposure. Mutations of the nuclear or mitochondrial genome may be causative, or at least contributive. Interestingly, mutations of the mitochondrial genome may appear spontaneously (possibly caused by toxin and/or radiation exposure), blurring the boundary between genetic and environmental causes. Mitochondrial dysfunction may lead to oxidative stress, proteasomal overload, protein aggregation, and changes in neuronal firing properties. Most important of all, however, is energy (adenosine 5'-triphosphate, ATP) depletion, as energy supply is the primary cellular function of mitochondria. Thus, therapies aimed at correcting this energy deficit, such as creatine or coenzyme Q_{10}, have shown promise in exploratory neuroprotection trials in PD (see Chapter 2).

c. Mechanisms of cell death in Parkinson's disease: therapeutic implications

In the substantia nigra of PD patients, dopaminergic neurons can be divided into three groups: (1) normal neurons, (2) diseased neurons, and (3) dying neurons (Fig. 1.11). One of the major questions over the past decade has been whether dopaminergic (and possibly other) neurons in PD die by apoptosis (programmed cell death) or necrosis.

Programmed cell death was long considered identical to apoptosis but has been shown to encompass other forms of cell death such as autophagy. In theory, programmed cell death is an attractive candidate for drug therapy in PD for two reasons. First, specific molecular pathways are engaged to induce degradation of intracellular constituents and, ultimately, phagocytosis of the cell. These molecular pathways can be targeted pharmacologically. Second, programmed cell death is the common endpoint and thus denominator for multiple pathogenic processes leading to cell death. Since programmed cell death in PD, however, seems to be a consequence of cellular dysfunction rather than a primary disease phenomenon, questions

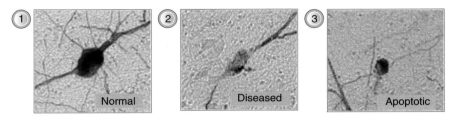

Figure 1.11 Mechanisms of neuronal death in Parkinson's disease. Dopaminergic neurons in Parkinson's disease can be found in three states: (1) Normal. Neurons display strong tyrosine hydroxylase (TH) staining, indicative of dopamine content. The neuron has several dentrites and a well-developed axon. (2) Diseased. The cell body begins to shrink. TH staining is weak and dentrites/axons begin to retract. (3) Dying (apoptotic). The nucleus is condensed, and the cell body maximally shrunken. TH staining is weak or absent, and dentrites/axons are completely retracted.

have been raised whether it represents a worthwhile therapeutic target. The major concern relates to whether programmed cell death inhibition is sufficient to protect *and* restore function of neurons in PD. This is probably not the case. Rather, it is plausible to assume that programmed cell death inhibition will result in the survival of *diseased* neurons, while treatment should aim at restoring these cells (Fig. 1.12).

Therefore, therapeutic interventions to rescue diseased neurons must target pathways upstream of the molecular cascade regulating programmed cell death. Before undergoing programmed cell death, a dopaminergic neuron

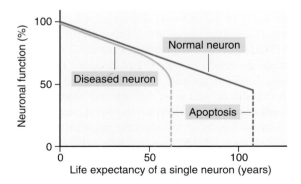

Figure 1.12 Function of a dopaminergic neuron during normal aging and in Parkinson's disease. When apoptosis occurs, neuronal function has already significantly declined. Thus, while anti-apoptotic therapies may "rescue" sick neurons, they fail to restore adequate function.

does not degenerate abruptly (although the exact kinetics in humans remain unknown), but crosses several intermediate stages, possibly over the course of years. This means that a proportion of neurons may be suffering and dysfunctional, but morphologically intact. Early rescue of diseased neurons may clinically result in an improvement in symptoms or, with the prospect of future preclinical identification of PD, delay the symptomatic phase of the disease and halt its progression.

One of the main problems, however, is to understand what the *causes* and the *consequences* of the primary disease process ("sporadic," genetic, and/or environmental) are. Indeed, it is extremely difficult to disentangle the primary from the secondary events in this cascade, where all intracellular pathophysiological alterations potentially interact. Once neuronal suffering occurs, multiple pathways are probably engaged in *parallel* and not sequentially. This means that a neuroprotective/neurorestorative treatment should probably target as many pathways as possible ("cocktail approach") instead of relying on a single, highly specific "magic bullet."

Further reading
Abeliovich A, Flint Beal M. Parkinsonism genes: culprits and clues. *J Neurochem* 2006; **99**(4): 1062–72.
Benmoyal-Segal L, Soreq H. Gene-environment interactions in sporadic Parkinson's disease. *J Neurochem* 2006; **97**(6): 1740–55.
Hardy J, Cai H, Cookson MR, Gwinn-Hardy K, Singleton A. Genetics of Parkinson's disease and parkinsonism. *Ann Neurol* 2006; **60**(4): 389–98.
Hartmann A. Programmed cell death in Parkinson's disease. In: *Recent Breakthroughs in Basal Ganglia Research*, Ed. Bezard E. New York: Nova Science Publishers, 2006: 303–12.
Sulzer D. Multiple hit hypotheses for dopamine neuron loss in Parkinson's disease. *Trends Neurosci* 2007; **30**(5): 244–50.
Schapira AHV. Mitochondria in the aetiology and pathogenesis of Parkinson's disease. *Lancet Neurol* 2008; **7**(1): 97–109.

5. Conclusions
a. Parkinson's disease or Parkinson's *syndromes*?
Despite decades of intense research, the etiology of PD remains unknown. One fundamental point which has begun to emerge over the past decade, however, is that PD is not a single entity. Both environmental agents and genetic causes as well as age-related effects have been identified with potentially important interactions. In particular, the discovery of Mendelian forms of PD are challenging the concept that PD is one disease, as well as the validity of the current clinicopathological disease definition.

Another important paradigm shift in our understanding of PD concerns non-motor symptoms. Clinicians involved in the care of PD patients have known for a long time that this disorder comprises far more than the classic motor triad of symptoms (akinesia/bradykinesia, rigidity, and rest tremor, see below). Rather, a multitude of non-motor symptoms either co-occur with the motor triad, appear later in the disease course, or may even *precede* the motor triad. The underlying neuropathological and neurochemical central nervous system alterations explaining these symptoms are just beginning to be identified, however, and their treatment is complex.

Finally, it is important to understand that the cellular dysfunctions leading to cell death observed in PD brains occur gradually. Thus, the nigrostriatal dopaminergic system and other systems may be dysfunctional, although morphologically intact at the perikaryal, axonal, and/or synaptic level. This has major therapeutic implications, since rescue of these neurons may well suffice to achieve adequate clinical improvement, potentially without additional symptomatic therapies being required.

Thus, the holy grail of PD research is to stop disease progression by protecting healthy neurons (neuroprotection) or even reverse the disease course by restoring the function of diseased neurons (neurorescue). Both patients and the medical community express the same priority, despite or maybe even because of the availability of multiple efficient symptomatic treatments (see Chapter 2).

b. What Parkinson's disease is not

In light of these observations, however, it is also helpful to recall what PD *is not*:

• *PD is a multisystem, but not a generalized disease of the brain:* Although many different neuronal populations may be involved, especially in late disease

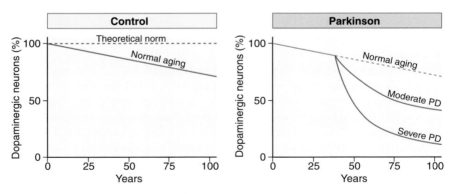

Figure 1.13 The temporal pattern of dopaminergic cell loss in Parkinson's disease. Whereas in normal aging, a slow and steady decline in the number of dopaminergic neurons occurs, this decline is much sharper in Parkinson's disease (variable, either relatively slow in some forms of the disease, or abrupt in severe cases), beginning (presumably) in middle age for the classic forms of the disease.

stages, the majority of neurons in the central nervous system remain undamaged.

• *PD is not an accelerated form of aging:* Although neuronal death probably occurs slowly (both at the systemic and at the cellular level), the decline is still much sharper than during normal aging (Fig. 1.13). Thus, it is estimated that nigral neuronal loss is 1% per year in PD patients, while neuronal loss with aging may be minimal, although connectivity and cellular function do decline. Furthermore, the type and localization of neurons most affected by PD or by aging differ. Thus, cell loss is more pronounced in the ventral tier of the substantia nigra in PD, whereas in normal aging, loss that does occur affects the dorsal tier. Finally, the recognition of juvenile forms of PD contradicts the notion that PD is necessarily an age-related disease.

• *PD is not an embryopathy:* Although the precise moment when neuronal degeneration starts is unknown, nuclear imaging data have provided compelling evidence that the neuronal loss (but not necessarily subclinical neuronal dysfunction) begins in adulthood. Moreover, the period between the onset of neuronal loss and the appearance of clinical symptoms probably spans less than a decade.

• *PD is not a well-defined, consensual entity:* Although both clinical and histopathological criteria for PD exist, familial forms have shed doubt on the validity of these criteria. In addition, the renewed interest in non-dopaminergic lesions in PD, which may even precede the onset of the parkinsonian motor triad, has triggered a debate to what extent the multisystemic nature of PD must be taken into account when formulating diagnostic criteria.

In conclusion, PD consists of dopaminergic lesions, both cerebral and extracerebral, and non-dopaminergic cerebral lesions. The extent and evolution of these lesions varies greatly from patient to patient. Although the Braak staging is an elegant attempt to provide a general frame for the evolution of lesions and symptoms, it is merely a model that does not suffice to predict individual prognosis. Rather, there is still progress to be made in semiology which remains, by and large, the best reflection of brain function. Thus, the different clinical features of PD will be addressed in the following section and correlated with the underlying pathophysiology.

II. Clinical features of Parkinson's disease

1. Motor symptoms

To diagnose PD requires identifying parkinsonism first. Parkinsonism is characterized by akinesia and rigidity, of which idiopathic ("sporadic") PD is the main cause. PD is a clinical and neuropathological entity (loss of pigmented dopaminergic neurons in the brain stem, particularly in the sustantia nigra along with the presence of Lewy bodies) that is included within the spectrum of parkinsonism. In theory, therefore, the only way to confirm a diagnosis of

PD is by autopsy. Nevertheless, patient history and examination by skilled clinicians can predict the pathological findings with high certainty. PD is usually asymmetrical, characterized by the presence of akinesia and rigidity, often associated with rest tremor, and is responsive to dopaminergic treatment. Furthermore, historical or examination factors suggesting an alternative cause for symptoms are lacking (Table 1.5).

The cardinal feature of parkinsonism remains *akinesia,* that is a difficulty in *initiating* a movement, which can be measured by increased reaction time. *Bradykinesia* or slowing of movements is less specific than akinesia. *Hypometria* or incomplete movement is revealed by alternate movements of the extremities. In addition, sequential movements (for instance drinking, which associates grasping a glass followed by flexion of the elbow) or concomitant movements (executing two movements at the same time in different limbs) are altered. Moreover, akinesia is also influenced by decreased motivation and mood and is thus a complex symptom whose origin is not strictly sensorimotor. In clinical practice, these symptoms are revealed by reduced arm swing when walking, micrographia, and difficult execution of fine movements (e.g. fishing a coin out of a pocket). The patient's face is unexpressive, walking is slow, and the feet are not raised sufficiently.

Rigidity is not a symptom but a sign. It is detectable in distal joints (for instance the wrist). If present in proximal joints, the neck and/or the trunk, prognosis is worrying since axial rigidity does not respond as well to dopa-

Table 1.5 Clinical diagnostic criteria for Parkinson's disease

Clinically possible	**Exclusion criteria**
One of:	• Exposure to drugs that can cause
• asymmetric resting tremor (4–6 Hz; 70%	parkinsonism, such as neuroleptics, some
of PD patients)	anti-emetic drugs, tetrabenazine, reserpine,
• asymmetric rigidity	flunarizine and cinnarizine
• asymmetric bradykinesia	• Cerebellar signs
	• Corticospinal tract signs
Clinically probable	• Eye-movement abnormalities other than
Any two of:	slight limitation of upward gaze
• asymmetric resting tremor	• Severe dysautonomia
• asymmetric rigidity	• Early moderate to severe gait disturbance or
• asymmetric bradykinesia	dementia
	• History of encephalitis, recurrent head injury
Clinically definite	(such as seen in boxers)
Criteria for clinically probable, plus:	• Evidence of severe subcortical white-
• substantial and sustained response to	matter disease, hydrocephalus or other
antiparkinson drugs	structural lesions on MRI that may account for
	parkinsonism

Samii A, *et al. Lancet* 2004; **363**: 1783–94; Calne DB, *et al. Ann Neurol* 1992; **32**(Suppl): S125–7; Ward CD, Gibb WR. *Adv Neurol* 1990; **53**: 245–9.

minergic treatment or may even indicate a Parkinson-plus syndrome. By nature, parkinsonian rigidity is plastic, often giving way in a series of small jerks ("cogwheel rigidity"). If subtle, rigidity can be increased following the Froment maneuver (active mobilization of the contralateral limb). Parkinsonian ("lead-pipe") rigidity must be distinguished from pyramidal ("clasp-knife") rigidity and oppositional rigidity ("gegenhalten"), the latter being provoked or increased by movements and owing to diffuse cerebral lesions.

Rest tremor is usually the first symptom noticed by the patient, although it can occasionally be absent. It is regular (4–6 Hz frequency) and increases with emotional and mental stress (e.g. counting backwards). Rest tremor is usually most visible when the patient is walking, and does not always disappear during posture or action when it is, however, weaker than at rest.

Postural instability, sometimes considered a cardinal symptom, is non-specific and absent early on in the disease, particularly in younger patients. If present, it is often the consequence of non-dopaminergic brain lesions, as seen in patients with Parkinson-plus syndromes (see below).

The three cardinal PD symptoms respond well to levodopa therapy, since they result from the degeneration of the nigrostriatal dopaminergic pathway. Their pathophysiology is not entirely understood. Bradykinesia is considered to result from the demodulation of striato-pallido-thalamo-frontal circuits by the damaged nigrostriatal dopaminergic system. Rigidity has the same origin, but additional dysfunction of neuronal pathways connecting the basal ganglia to lower brain structures has been hypothesized. Parkinsonian rest tremor is equally of basal ganglia origin, since its characteristic frequency can be detected in these structures. However, a cerebellar component is also probably involved, as suggested by the spectacular improvement of tremor by lesioning the cerebellar relay of the thalamus following stereotactic neurosurgery.

Motor symptoms in advanced PD patients, however, can also result from non-dopaminergic lesions. These symptoms are called "axial" because they evolve around the body's central axis. Nine typical axial symptoms can be distinguished: memory impairment (subcorticofrontal syndrome), abnormal ocular movements, nuchal rigidity, dysarthria, swallowing difficulties, posture abnormalities, sphincter problems, postural instability, and abnormal gait. Looking out for these symptoms is an integral part of the examination of patients presenting with parkinsonism (Table 1.6). In addition, autonomic symptoms – sexual dysfunction, constipation, orthostatic hypotension, seborrhea – and sleep disturbances may be present. If doubts persist, four tests may contribute to the diagnosis: (1) neuropsychological examination; (2) ocular movement recording, (3) cystomanometry; (4) brain MRI.

Table 1.6 How to examine a Parkinson's disease (PD) patient. When examining a PD patient, 20 items (in four parts) can be used to obtain a complete assessment

Assessment	Items
History	Age, symptom onset, type and localization of first symptom(s), family history of PD
Parkinsonian syndrome	Akinesia/bradykinesia, rigidity, rest tremor
Effect of dopaminergic/dopamimetic therapy	Efficacy, dyskinesia, motor fluctuations, psychiatric side effects (visual hallucinations)
"Axial" symptoms	

Further reading

Tolosa E, Wenning G, Poewe W. The diagnosis of Parkinson's disease. *Lancet Neurol* 2006; 5(1): 75–86.

2. Non-motor symptoms

The excellent control of parkinsonian motor symptoms provided by dopaminergic therapies and functional neurosurgery means that it is now common to see patients with disease progression over a period of 15–20 years or even longer. As a result, non-motor symptoms seem to occur more frequently in advanced PD patients. These symptoms, which may also appear early or even precede the characteristic parkinsonian motor features, include psychiatric symptoms (depression, anxiety, apathy, cognitive impairment); sleep disorders; autonomic symptoms (cardiovascular system, gut, and bladder) and sensory symptoms (Table 1.7). Even though these non-motor symptoms are

Table 1.7 Non-motor symptoms

Neuropsychiatric symptoms	Gastrointestinal symptoms
Depression, anxiety	Drooling
Apathy	Dysphagia and choking
Anhedonia	Nausea (can be drug-induced)
Attention deficit	Constipation
Hallucinations, illusions, delusions (can be drug-induced)	Unsatisfactory voiding of bowel
Dementia	
Obsessional behavior (can be drug-induced) and repetitive	**Sensory symptoms**
behavior	Pain
Confusion (can be drug-induced)	Paresthesia
	Olfactory disturbance
Sleep disorders	
Restless legs and periodic limb movements	**Other symptoms**
Rapid eye movement (REM) sleep behavior disorder	Fatigue
Excessive daytime somnolence	Diplopia
Sudden onset of sleep ("sleep attacks")	Blurred vision
Insomnia	Seborrhea
Autonomic symptoms	
Bladder disturbances	
Sweating	
Orthostatic hypotension	
Sexual dysfunction (erectile impotence)	
Hypersexuality (likely to be drug-induced)	

frequently the ones that trouble patients the most and contribute significantly to morbidity and impaired quality of life, they are often insufficiently recognized and inadequately treated.

a. Depression

Depression is the most common psychiatric symptom of PD, and is a major determinant of poor quality of life. It is said that some 50% of early PD patients suffer from depression, many even before the appearance of motor symptoms. A significant biological rather than a purely reactive basis for depression associated with PD is thus highly probable (Chapter 3, case study 12).

The clinical profile of PD depression is characterized by depressed mood and loss of motivation and initiative, anhedonia, anxiety, panic attacks, loss of appetite, and social withdrawal. Suicidal ideation, self-reproach, and feelings of guilt are less common, however. This explains why most depressed PD patients fulfill criteria for minor depression or dysthymic disorder rather than for major depression.

Depression can occur in patients who have been treated with suboptimal doses of dopaminergic treatment that keep them in a prolonged "off" period, usually associated with painful dystonia and anxiety. More frequently, however, depressive states in PD patients result from the dysfunction of dopaminergic, noradrenergic, and serotonergic neuronal systems. Since there is a clear dopaminergic effect on mood and anxiety, dopaminergic supply (via levodopa or dopamine agonists) represents the first-line treatment of parkinsonian depression. The mechanism of action of levodopa and dopamine agonists may involve the stimulation of dopamine receptors located in limbic areas of the basal ganglia and the cerebral cortex. This also means, however, that hypomania can sometimes be observed when patients are overtreated with dopaminergic agents, especially dopamine agonists. Moreover, there is a constant although partial degeneration in PD of noradrenergic and serotonergic neurons (originating respectively in the locus coeruleus and raphe nucleus). Dysfunction of these neuronal systems is known to play a role in depression. Therefore, treatment with serotonin and/or noradrenaline reuptake inhibitors, which reestablish normal concentrations of noradrenaline and serotonin in limbic brain areas, are used in most depressed PD patients in addition to baseline dopaminergic treatment.

b. Apathy

Apathy, which can be summarized as decreased motivation, has now been established as a distinctive symptom of PD independent of depression and fatigue. The features of apathy in PD do not respond to dopaminergic drugs in all patients, possibly indicating more extensive contributions from other neurotransmitter systems.

c. Cognitive impairment

It is estimated that about 40% of all PD patients develop dementia, a rate about six times higher than that in healthy individuals matched for age. Whereas severe cognitive impairment is observed late during the disease, subtle cognitive alterations are common even in early PD, mainly affecting frontal executive functions (Chapter 3, case study 14). Intellectual impairment in patients can be subdivided into two categories: subcortical and cortical.

1 The slight cognitive alterations seen early during the course of the disease are usually of the "subcortical" type, characterized by a dysexecutive syndrome, including attention deficits, cognitive slowing and decreased concentration abilities. Moderate memory impairment can be observed, defined by a retrieval deficit rather than an impairment in information storage. It is not always easy to differentiate such frontal lobe-like symptomatology from depression. In clinical practice, such distinction is important since the treatment of depression and cognitive impairment is different. These symptoms result from the "demodulation" of prefrontal areas as a result of the progressive degeneration of subcortical neurons, including the long ascending dopaminergic (ventral tegmental area), cholinergic (nucleus basalis of Meynert), noradrenergic (locus coeruleus), and serotonergic (raphe nucleus) systems. In patients in whom a dysexecutive syndrome or depression is suspected, various neuropsychological tests are of interest in clinical practice to distinguish them from full-blown dementia (Table 1.8). This cognitive profile is characteristic enough to distinguish cognitive impairment in PD patients from that found

Table 1.8 Proposed neuropsychological battery to diagnose movement disorders

	Test	Assessment
Dementia	Mattis Dementia Rating Scale	"Subcortico-frontal" dementia
Memory	California Verbal Learning Test	Strategic learning impairment in non-demented patients
	Grober and Buschke Test	Distinguish retrieval deficits from genuine amnesia in demented patients
Instrumental functions		
Language	Boston Diagnostic Aphasia Examination	Differentiate true aphasia from lexical evocation deficits using at least the naming and comprehension subtests
Gesture	Apraxia examination	Single out true apraxia using at least the imitation of symbolic gestures and actual utilization of objects
Executive functions		Detect a frontal lobe-like syndrome
Sorting	Wisconsin Card Sorting Test	
Fluency	Lexical fluency	
Series	Graphic and motor series	
Interference	Stroop Test	
Shifting	Trail Making Test	
Behaviors	Prehension, utilization, imitation	

Based on Pillon B, Dubois B, Agid Y. Testing cognition may contribute to the diagnosis of movement disorders. *Neurology* 1996; **46**(2): 331.

in other parkinsonian disorders such as progressive supranuclear palsy, corticobasal degeneration and dementia with Lewy bodies (Table 1.9). This is not the case for multiple system atrophy, however, since the pattern of intellectual impairment is identical to that of PD.

2 Beside these slowly evolving cognitive difficulties of "subcortical" origin, an authentic dementia of cortical origin can occur in PD patients, usually at end-stage disease (Chapter 3, case study 20). The clinical picture of dementia consists of a severe memory disorder: here, not only the retrieval of information is altered, but also its storage. This cortical memory impairment is not associated with other cognitive symptoms of cortical origin such as seen in Alzheimer's disease; language, praxic, and gnosic capabilities are spared. Cortical dementia comprises disseminated neuronal losses in the cerebral cortex associated with various histopathological stigmata, namely neurofibrillar tangles and/or Lewy bodies. The debate whether PD plus dementia and dementia with Lewy bodies form separate entities or are located within the same disease spectrum is still ongoing. Clinically, they seem to be undistinguishable (Table 1.10) although dementia and visual hallucinations are seen early during the course of the disease in patients with Lewy body disease.

In sum, most patients with PD remain intellectually intact. If present, cognitive impairment evolves in two steps during the course of the disease. A first period is characterized by slight to moderate frontal subcortical cognitive impairment which remains isolated for several years, followed by the occurrence

Table 1.9 Neuropsychological pattern in patients with movement disorders

	PD	MSA	CBD	PSP	PDD	HD	DLBD	AD+EP
Dementia								
Global impairment	–	–	–	+	+	+	+	++
Fluctuations	–	–	–	–	–	–	+	–
Memory								
Storage disorders	–	–	–	–	–	–	+	++
Recall disorders	+	+	+	++	++	++	+	+
Instrumental disorders								
Linguistic	–	–	+	±	±	±	+	++
Praxic	–	–	++	±	±	±	+	+
Executive disorders								
Planning	+	+	+	++	++	+	+	+
Behavior	±	±	+	++	+	±	±	±
Psychosis	–	–	–	–	±	+	++	+

Abbreviations: PD, Parkinson's disease; MSA, multiple system atrophy; CBD, corticobasal degeneration; PSP, progressive supranuclear palsy; PDD, Parkinson's disease with dementia; HD, Huntington's disease; DLBD, diffuse Lewy body disease; AD+EP, Alzheimer's disease plus extrapyramidal signs.

- = absent; ± = mild or discussed; + = moderate or present in a proportion of patients; ++ = severe and present in a majority of patients. Highlighting underlines the neuropsychological characteristics of each disease.

Pillon B, Dubois B, Agid Y. *Neurology* 1996; **46**(2): 331.

Table 1.10 Features of Parkinson's disease plus dementia and dementia with Lewy bodies

Dementia is mild to moderate compared to Alzheimer's disease
Insight is usually preserved
Impaired attention with fluctuations: these patients are better in the morning and worse in the evening
Impaired executive functions
Impaired internally-cued behavior
Impaired memory: these patients can store information, but have problems accessing it
Poor visual-spatial function
Language by and large is intact
Prominent behavioral symptoms which include frequent delusions, hallucinations, and mood and personality changes

of true cortical dementia in a minor proportion of patients. Whatever the type of cognitive disability, the symptomatic treatment of intellectual disturbances is difficult, since most drugs are inefficacious. Nevertheless, the use of cholinesterase inhibitors can be helpful since cholinergic cell loss in the nucleus basalis of Meynert, resulting in severe cholinergic demodulation of the cerebral cortex, has been described in advanced demented PD patients.

d. Sleep

The prevalence of sleep disorders in PD patients is probably superior to 75%. Most if not all patients suffer from insomnia. The causes of insomnia are multifactorial. Nocturnal akinesia, often associated with painful dystonia (usually during bouts of severe anxiety), is a major contributive factor.

REM sleep behavior disorder is a pathological sleep structure (parasomnia) characterized by the loss of REM sleep muscle atonia, allowing patients to physically act out their dreams which are often violent. Bed partners commonly complain of vocalizations (talking, shouting, threats) and abnormal movements (waving arms or legs about, falling out of bed, violent outbursts). Whether REM sleep behavior disorder may ultimately serve as a preclinical marker for PD remains to be demonstrated, but it is now well established that REM sleep behavior disorder precedes the appearance of parkinsonian motor features in up to a third of patients (Chapter 3, case studies 1 and 6).

Excessive daytime sleepiness affects up to 50% of PD patients. It is probably caused by a combination of the disease process, the effect of nocturnal sleep disruption, and antiparkinsonian drugs including levodopa and dopamine agonists. In these patients, sleep latency is severely reduced ($<5\,min$) and episodes of sudden-onset sleep are often observed. The occurrence of sudden-onset sleep must be taken very seriously, since it interferes with the ability of patients to drive.

To ascertain diagnosis of sleep disorders, polysomnography may be helpful (i) to quantify the length of insomnia periods, (ii) to evaluate potential dangers derived from daytime sleepiness and sudden-onset sleep, and (iii) to confirm the existence and the semiology of REM sleep behavior disorder.

The causes of these sleep disorders are still a matter of debate. Degeneration of central sleep regulation centers in the brainstem (pedunculopontine nucleus and nucleus subcoeruleus) and dysfunction of thalamocortical pathways have been implicated in the pathogenesis of these sleep disorders. Furthermore, the loss of hypocretin-containing neurons in the hypothalamus very likely contribute to the occurrence of narcolepsy-like episodes.

e. Autonomic dysfunction
Contrary to previous beliefs, cardiovascular dysfunction, which includes orthostatic hypotension and increased heart rate at rest, may occur early in the disease. This results mainly from reduced sympathetic noradrenergic innervation of the heart and baroreflex failure (nucleus vagus lesions). Symptoms only tend to become severe in late disease stages, however. Treatment with dopaminergic agents (which induce peripheral vasodilation) may exacerbate orthostatic hypotension, but is rarely the main contributor.

Gastrointestinal dysfunction manifests as impaired swallowing, impaired gastric motility and, most bothersome to PD patients, constipation. Degeneration of dopaminergic neurons in the mesenteric plexus, causing colonic sympathetic denervation, is one of the underlying mechanisms for constipation. Constipation does not respond well to dopaminergic treatment, however, suggesting that non-dopaminergic mechanisms are also implicated.

Urogenital symptoms include impaired bladder function, leading to urinary emergencies and incontinence. Patients suffer either from a hypoactive bladder or, more frequently, from a hyperactive bladder. The latter is correlated with ni-grostriatal denervation, since physiological basal ganglia output has an overall inhibitory effect on the micturition reflex, which is decreased in PD.

Sexual dysfunction affects up to two-thirds of PD patients. As a direct consequence of the disease process, erectile dysfunction may occur. Although libido can be reduced, it can also be enhanced by antiparkinsonian dopaminergic medications, in particular by dopamine agonists. This can result in hypersexuality, which is part of the "dopaminergic dysregulation syndrome" (see below).

f. Sensory symptoms

Various types of abnormal sensations, most importantly pain, can be observed in advanced PD patients. Sensory symptoms can be distinguished into painful cramps related to "off"-period dystonia, and diffuse painful sensations also usually associated with "off" periods. The cerebral structures involved in altered pain processing are poorly characterized, but may comprise mesencephalic dopaminergic projections to the caudal thalamus.

Further reading
Chaudhuri KR, Healy DG, Schapira AH; National Institute for Clinical Excellence. Non-motor symptoms of Parkinson's disease: diagnosis and management. *Lancet Neurol* 2006; **5**(3): 235–45.

Emre M. Dementia associated with Parkinson's disease. *Lancet Neurol* 2003; **2**(4): 229–37.

Goldstein DS. Dysautonomia in Parkinson's disease: neurocardiological abnormalities. *Lancet Neurol* 2003; **2**(11): 669–76.

3. The different forms of Parkinson's disease: relevance for prognosis

Numerous studies have attempted to define prognostic factors for PD. All of these studies were retrospective, however, and only two factors have clearly emerged as valid to prognose progression of disability: higher age at disease onset and the occurrence of postural instability. The clinician, nevertheless, is often confronted with the understandable wish of patients and their families to estimate disease prognosis. From a practical perspective, several factors would seem to be helpful in anticipating the course of the disease:

1 *The rate of symptom progression* can be estimated during the patient's interview by calculating the approximate ratio between the severity of motor symptoms and the period of time elapsed since the appearance of the first symptom (Fig. 1.14).

2 *The detection of axial signs* always indicates a bad prognosis. At early disease stages, axial signs point towards Parkinson-plus syndromes. In advanced forms of PD, axial signs become the source of substantial handicaps, as they are poorly responsive or unresponsive to dopaminergic replacement therapy.

3 *The response of patients to levodopa* treatment is a key factor for the prognosis. At the beginning of the disease, a dramatic response to levodopa treatment will very likely lead to severe levodopa-induced motor complications. Even

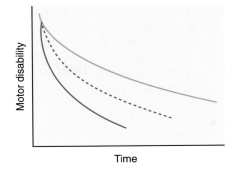

Figure 1.14 Rate of progression. The rate of symptom progression can be hypothesized in individual patients.

more alarming is a poor or absent response to levodopa treatment. Assessment of a patient's levodopa response may require several weeks of levodopa exposure, eventually using high dosages of the drug (up to 1000 mg/day) to exclude Parkinson-plus syndromes (Fig. 1.15).

4 *Good prognostic factors also include:* the absence of a proximal lead-pipe rigidity; the absence of early morning painful foot dystonia; and the absence of parkinsonian symptoms in the morning before the first dose of medication.

5 In difficult cases, a *brain MRI* can be useful, in particular in patients who respond poorly to levodopa replacement therapy. The prime role of imaging in PD is to exclude Parkinson-plus syndromes (severe enlargement of the third ventricle, cerebellar atrophy, severe atrophy of the mesencephalon, focal atrophy of the cerebral cortex). Non-degenerative features such as ventricular dilatation, lacunes, and diffuse white matter lesions can explain diminished response to dopaminergic treatment, and thereby indicate an unfavorable prognosis.

Further reading

Post B, Merkus MP, de Haan RJ *et al.* Prognostic factors for the progression of Parkinson's disease: a systematic review. *Mov Disord* 2007; **22**(13): 1839–51.

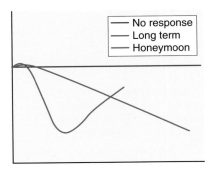

Figure 1.15 Response to levodopa treatment.

4. The differential diagnosis of Parkinson's disease

While PD is the most common cause of parkinsonism (defined as an akineto-rigid syndrome) and represents approximately 75% of cases, the remaining 25% may have multiple causes (Fig. 1.16). These parkinsonian patients pose a considerable diagnostic problem and, ultimately, a therapeutic challenge to the clinician, depending upon whether parkinsonism results from degenerative or non-degenerative lesions.

The most important differential diagnosis to PD to be considered are illnesses that can be cured; these are, however, extremely rare (Chapter 3, case study 3). Epidemiologically, essential tremor is the most common differential diagnosis for PD patients with tremor (Table 1.11). Typical essential tremor is characterized by bilateral, usually symmetrical, visible and persistent upper limb postural and/or kinetic tremor. The presence of a head or voice tremor, a robust autosomal dominant family history, and improvement with alcohol all favor the diagnosis of essential tremor. In contrast, a clear asymmetry of tremor, the selective involvement of the lower extremities, and the presence of bradykinesia or rigidity support a diagnosis of PD. The duration of symptoms is different: several years to decades in essential tremor, far less in PD. If doubts persist, nuclear imaging of dopaminergic terminals using single positron emission computed tomography (SPECT) with a dopamine transporter ligand can distinguish essential tremor from PD (Chapter 3, cases studies 2 and 16).

Drug-induced parkinsonism is most commonly induced by antipsychotic neuroleptic drugs that selectively block dopaminergic neurotransmission. These causes can easily be identified through a precise interview. It is important to bear in mind that patients are often also treated with other medications

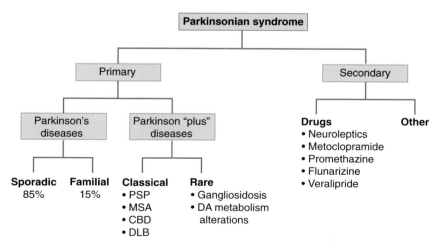

Figure 1.16 A decision tree for the differential diagnosis of parkinsonian syndromes. PSP, progressive supranuclear palsy; MSA, multiple system atrophy; CBD, corticobasal degeneration; DLB, dementia with Lewy bodies.

Table 1.11 Parkinson's disease and essential tremor: differential diagnosis

	Parkinson's disease	Essential tremor
Family history	Usually negative	Positive in the majority of cases
Usual patient's complaint	Dysfunction resulting from their various disabilities	Tremor
Alcohol intake	May reduce the tremor	Marked tremor reduction
Tremor type	Resting	Postural, kinetic
Body part affected	Hands, legs[a]	Hands, head, voice
Disease course	Progressive over months	Slowly progressive but with many periods of stasis, over years and decades
Bradykinesia, rigidity, postural instability	May be present	Never present
Tremor amplitude and frequency	4–6 Hz: slower than essential tremor, constant amplitude[b]	6–12 Hz: slightly faster than PD, varying amplitude
Treatment test		
Levodopa	Effective	No effect
Propranolol	May decrease tremor	Effective
Primidone	No effect	Effective

[a]While head tremor is unusual in PD, parkinsonian tremor can also affect legs, lips, jaw, and tongue, either alone or in combination with tremors of other body parts.
[b]Tremor in PD is commonly described as "pill rolling" because of a unique, 4–6 Hz rhythmic oscillation of flexion and extension movements of the thumb and fingers compared to the style of early pharmacists who rolled hand-made pills into little balls by using the thumb and forefinger.

that can block dopaminergic neurotransmission. These include anxiolytics, anti-nausea drugs, calcium channel blockers, and dopamine-depleting drugs (tetrabenazine). Drug-induced parkinsonism is classically characterized by symmetry of symptoms, absence of tremor, and lack of response to dopaminergic treatment, but slight asymmetry is often present. In the case of isolated parkinsonian features without a clear drug history, diagnosis of drug-induced parkinsonism can be challenging. Upon closer inspection, however, other symptoms may be associated, such as acathisia, freezing gait, facial dyskinesia or axial dystonia, favoring the diagnosis of tardive dyskinesia.

Table 1.12 gives other rare causes of parkinsonisms that also should be considered. In these cases, clinicians need to be attentive to atypical features in the history and during the examination of patients (Chapter 3, case studies 4, 5, 17, 19 and 23).

Table 1.12 Treatable/curable causes of parkinsonism

Wilson's disease
Hypoparathyroidism
Whipple's disease
Drug-induced: neuroleptics, lithium, reserpin, tetrabenazin, flunarizin, cinnarizin, amphetamines
Brain tumors
Toxin-induced: manganese, carbon monoxide, 1-methyl 4-phenyl 1,2,3,6-tetrahydropyridine (MPTP)
Encephalitis

The most frequent differential diagnosis of PD, however, are Parkinson-plus syndromes. These include corticobasal degeneration, multiple system atrophy, progressive supranuclear palsy, and dementia with Lewy bodies. When examining a patient with parkinsonism, the clinician regularly faces this problem as approximately 10% of patients who have received an initial clinical diagnosis of PD are ultimately found to have Parkinson-plus syndromes. Significantly diminished or absent response to levodopa treatment in these disorders occurs because of degeneration of striatal neurons and the resulting absence of postsynaptic dopamine receptors. These lesions, located downstream from lost dopaminergic nerve terminals ("in series" to the primary lesion) (Fig. 1.17), explain the severity of these neurodegenerative syndromes which cannot benefit from efficacious substitutive treatments to the same extent as PD. Typical features of Parkinson-plus syndromes compared to PD are listed in Table 1.13 (Chapter 3, cases studies 7, 8, 15 and 25).

Further reading

Ahlskog JE. Diagnosis and differential diagnosis of Parkinson's disease and parkinsonism. *Parkinsonism Relat Disord* 2000; **7**(1): 63–70.

Schapira AHV. Parkinson's disease. In: Schapira AHV, ed. *Neurology and Clinical Neuroscience.* Boston, MA: Elsevier; 2006.

Tolosa E, Wenning G, Poewe W. The diagnosis of Parkinson's disease. *Lancet Neurol* 2006; **5**(1): 75–86.

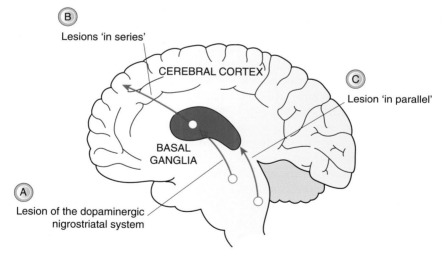

Figure 1.17 Brain lesions in patients with parkinsonism. The response to levodopa treatment depends on the presence of dopaminergic and non-dopaminergic lesions. When lesions only affect the nigrostriatal dopaminergic pathway (A), patients display an excellent levodopa response (15% of patients). When lesions occur postsynaptically of the nigrostriatal dopaminergic pathway (B), the levodopa response is poor or absent (15% of patients). When lesions occur in parallel to the nigrostriatal dopaminergic pathway (C), the levodopa response is intermediate (70% of patients). Adapted from Agid Y. Parkinson's disease: Pathophysiology. *Lancet* 1991;**337**:1321–24.

Table 1.13 Frequency of clinical characteristics in Parkinson's disease and in Parkinson-plus syndromes

	PD	DLB	MSA	PSP	CBD
Dementia		+			
Apraxia					+
Akinesia	+	+	+	+	+
Rigidity	+	+	+	+	+
Tremor	+	+			
Gait disturbances		+	+	+	+
Falls		+		+	+
Dysarthria		+	+	+	+
Dysphagia		+		+	
Gaze palsy				+	
Autonomic failure			+		

+, symptoms present in more than 70% of patients in postmortem series.
PD, Parkinson's disease; DLB, dementia with Lewy bodies; MSA, multisystem atrophy; PSP, progressive supranuclear palsy; CBD, corticobasal degeneration.
Adapted from Tolosa E, Wenning G, Poewe W. The diagnosis of Parkinson's disease. *Lancet Neurol* 2006; **5**(1): 75–86.

5. Treatment-related symptoms

a. Motor complications

Nowadays, PD is an eminently well-treatable neurological disorder. Yet, the available treatments also cause a multitude of side effects and complications that can profoundly affect quality of life and may require therapeutic solutions of their own.

Motor fluctuations are classically distinguished into two categories: (1) "wearing-off" periods during which levodopa-induced improvement in parkinsonian motor disability smoothly disappears at the end of action of a single dose of levodopa (Chapter 3, case study 9); and (2) "on-off" phenomena, i.e. motor fluctuations characterized by the abruptness with which immobility under levodopa treatment appears or disappears. Wearing-off phenomena correlate with the pharmacokinetics of levodopa. "On-off" phenomena require additional pharmacodynamic alterations, including sensitization of dopaminergic receptors (Chapter 3, case study 10). These changes reflect a gradual narrowing of the therapeutic window for levodopa as the disease progresses and daily treatment doses are increased. In advanced forms of PD, it may, therefore, become impossible to find a levodopa dose that has an antiparkinsonian effect without causing dyskinesias.

Dyskinesias develop at a rate of approximately 10% per annum, although this rate is much greater in young-onset PD patients, 70% of whom will develop dyskinesias within 3 years of levodopa initiation. Levodopa-induced dyskinesias can be subdivided into three types (Chapter 3, case studies 10 and 11):

1 *"Peak-dose" dyskinesias,* which occur most frequently, are choreatic and pre-dominant in the upper extremities. Patients, generally, do not feel particularly disabled by these dyskinesias, but consider them more as a social handicap.

2 *"Diphasic" dyskinesias,* which occur when the effect of levodopa either starts or ends, are dystonic and predominant in the lower extremities. They are often painful and thus disabling.

3 *"Off" dystonia,* which might be a variant of diphasic dyskinesias, is painful, predominates in the lower extremities, and occurs usually in the morning before taking the first dose of medication. In clinical practice, the different types of abnormal involuntary movements are often extremely difficult to assess as they are intermingled.

The pathophysiology of levodopa-induced dyskinesias is not entirely clear. It is generally admitted that three mechanisms contribute to the appearance of dykinesias: (1) loss of dopaminergic neurons within the nigrostriatal pathway: the severity of levodopa-induced dyskinesias correlates positively with loss of dopaminergic nerve terminals in the motor part of the striatum; (2) the priming (sensitization) of striatal dopamine receptors: following chronic levodopa treatment, these receptors become hypersensitive to stimulation. In contrast to the tolerance (desensitization) obtained with most drugs, the administration of levodopa induces an exaggerated motor response; (3) the mode of administration of levodopa during the disease course: this is both a function of the pulsatile administration of levodopa, and the amount of individual levodopa doses used. Given that none of the compounds tested to date have unequivocally demonstrated neuroprotective properties, all PD patients will require levodopa treatment sooner or later. Clinicians therefore have to modulate, as much as possible, the mode of administration of levodopa and its derivatives, the goal being to delay the introduction of levodopa as long as possible by early administration of dopamine agonists, and to administer the minimal dose of levodopa able to induce an optimal clinical benefit while avoiding the onset of motor side effects.

b. Non-motor complications

Neuropsychiatric symptoms in PD induced by dopaminergic therapy – especially high-dose dopamine agonist therapy – include euphoria, hypomania, hypersexuality, pathological gambling, punding (complex prolonged, purposeless, and stereotyped behavior), and dopamine dysregulation syndrome (self-medication and addiction to dopaminergic drugs) (Chapter 3, case study 18). Although there is little hard evidence at present, abnormality of dopamine regulation within the nucleus accumbens and increased activation of the mesolimbic reward system have been proposed as possible mechanisms.

Visual hallucinations in PD patients develop late in the disease course and are usually benign. The clinical phenomenology is characterized as a complex visual image occurring in the alert state with open eyes. More sinister symptoms such as delusions, paranoid ideation, and delirium may become more frequent as the disease progresses. Visual hallucinations have been commonly viewed as an adverse effect of antiparkinsonian treatment, especially follow-ing treatment with dopamine agonists. Factors such as disease severity, de-mentia, depression, and decreased visual acuity, however, are more important determinants for visual hallucinations than dosage or duration of antiparkin-sonian medication. Their treatment is difficult and sometimes disappointing. There are essentially three strategies which can be successively used: (1) adapt antiparkinsonian treatment, essentially to avoid dopamine agonists and to stop additional symptomatic treatment (e.g. amantadine or anticholinergics) which can cause hallucinations or confusion; (2) increase cholinergic trans-mission through the use of cholinesterase inhibitors which can improve visual hallucinations; and (3) in difficult cases, add atypical antipsychotics which have no extrapyramidal effects, such as clozapine.

Further reading
Cenci MA. Dopamine dysregulation of movement control in L-DOPA-induced dyskinesia. *Trends Neurosci* 2007; **30**(5): 236–43.
Pontone G, Williams JR, Bassett SS, Marsh L. Clinical features associated with impulse con-trol disorders in Parkinson disease. *Neurology* 2006; **67**(7): 1258–61.

2 | Treatment of Parkinson's disease

Anthony Schapira, Andreas Hartmann, Yves Agid

I. Antiparkinsonian agents

The treatment of Parkinson's disease (PD) comprises several stages determined by the natural progression of the disease and by the complications that can develop as a consequence of drug use (Fig. 2.1). Dopaminergic agents are the drugs that are most effective in improving the motor deficits of PD and include levodopa, dopamine agonists, and the monoamine oxidase B (MAO-B) inhibitors. Several new drugs will shortly be released and reflect the rapid increase in treatment options for PD.

Stage One

1. Signs and symptoms on one side only
2. Symptoms mild
3. Symptoms inconvenient but not disabling
4. Usually presents with tremor of one limb
5. Friends have noticed changes in posture, locomotion and facial expression

Stage Two

1. Symptoms are bilateral
2. Minimal disability
3. Posture and gait affected

Stage Three

1. Significant slowing of body movements
2. Early impairment of equilibrium on walking or standing
3. Generalized dysfunction that is moderately severe

Stage Four

1. Severe symptoms
2. Can still walk to a limited extent
3. Rigidity and bradykinesia
4. No longer able to live alone
5. Tremor may be less than earlier stages

Stage Five

1. Cachectic stage
2. Invalidism complete
3. Cannot stand or walk
4. Requires constant nursing care

Figure 2.1 Hoehn and Yahr staging of Parkinson's disease. (Hoehn MM, Yahr MD. Parkinsonism: onset, progression and mortality. *Neurology* 1967;**17**: 427-42.)

1. Levodopa

Levodopa was the first drug to be used to replace the dopamine deficiency of PD and remains the "gold standard" against which the efficacy of other drugs is judged. Only 1% of an oral dose of levodopa is absorbed into the blood because of extensive metabolism in the gut. Consequently, it is routinely combined with a dopa decarboxylase (DDC) inhibitor to reduce peripheral metabolism that in turn both increases absorption to 10% and decreases side effects. Dual inhibition of peripheral metabolism with a combination of both a DDC inhibitor and an inhibitor of catechol-O-methyltransferase (COMT) is now possible. Levodopa and other dopaminergic agents improve both the quality of life and life expectancy of PD patients. It provides rapid and effective relief of bradykinesia, rigidity, and associated pain, and improves tremor in many patients. Levodopa improves symptoms in early PD patients by 12 to 13 Unified Parkinson's Disease Rating Scale (UPDRS) points after 3 months.

Side effects are mainly gastrointestinal and comprise nausea, vomiting, and anorexia. These usually disappear over 2–3 weeks, but may persist in some patients. They can be prevented or treated with domperidone 10–20 mg t.i.d., taken usually for a period of 2–4 weeks.

Levodopa has a long duration response in early disease that enables adequate symptomatic control with dosage schedules of three times daily (Fig. 2.2). Disease progression and the direct pharmacological effects of levodopa erode its utility, however, as 70% of patients develop motor complications within 6 years of initiation of the drug. Wearing-off, the re-emergence of dopamine-related symptoms, frequently requires modification of dosage and/or dose frequency, or the introduction of additional or alternative therapies, e.g. COMT inhibition (see Chapter 3, case study 9). Interestingly, so long as the plasma levodopa concentration is maintained, the clinical response will persist; wearing-off does not occur if the drug is given by continuous infusion.

Another significant long-term complication of levodopa use is the development of dyskinesias which, together with wearing-off, constitute the motor complications caused by levodopa. Dyskinesias develop at a rate of approximately 10% per annum, although this rate is much greater in young-onset PD patients, 70% of whom will have dyskinesias within 3 years of levodopa initiation. The mechanisms by which these motor complications develop are not completely understood, but pulsatile stimulation of dopamine receptors by short-acting agents including levodopa, and the degree of striatal denervation have been implicated. Dyskinesias may occur at the time of maximal clinical benefit and peak concentration of levodopa (peak-dose dyskinesias) or appear at the onset and decline of the levodopa effect (diphasic dyskinesias). Motor complications can be an important source of disability for some patients who cycle between "on" periods which are complicated by dyskinesias and "off" periods in which they suffer severe parkinsonism (see Chapter 3, case studies 10 and 11).

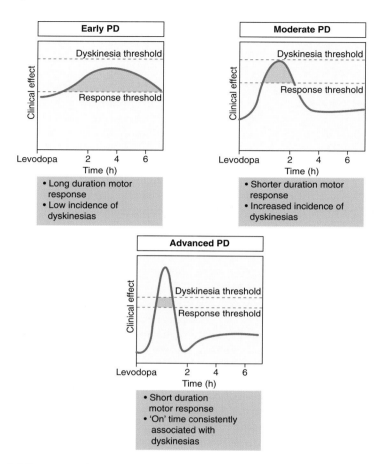

Figure 2.2 Response to levodopa and progression of Parkinson's disease. Treatment complications with levodopa. Early use of levodopa produces a long-duration response. With disease progression, this shortens and in clinical terms, patients begin to oscillate between being "on" with dyskinesias and being "off." The pharmacokinetics of levodopa do not change with disease progression, but the progress of the disease and the changes induced by levodopa produce downstream changes that are thought to induce the motor fluctuations. (Obeso JA, Olanow W, Nutt JG. Levodopa motor complications in Parkinson's disease. *Trends Neurosci* 2000;**23**(Suppl.):S2-7.)

Thus, levodopa offers a rapidly effective means to treat the motor symptoms of PD, with a tolerable early side-effect profile, but more serious long-term complications.

2. COMT inhibitors

The routine combination of levodopa with a DDC inhibitor improves absorption but the majority of levodopa is still metabolized in the gut by COMT which produces 3-*O*-methyldopa. COMT inhibition, therefore, offers a strat-

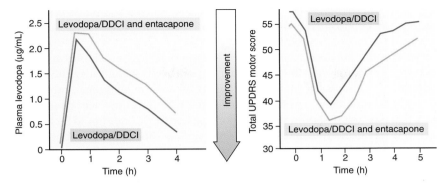

Figure 2.3 Strategies to improve levodopa delivery: effect of levodopa/dopa-decarboxylase inhibitor (DDCI) and entacapone on levodopa profile. COMT inhibition increases the half-life of levodopa and produces a parallel improvement in motor control.

egy to increase levodopa absorption and improve kinetics (Fig. 2.3). Two selective COMT inhibitors, entacapone and tolcapone, are available for clinical use for the treatment of PD. These drugs improve levodopa kinetics by increasing its bioavailability and elimination half-life. This allows more stable levodopa plasma levels to be obtained via the oral route and, conceivably, more sustained brain dopaminergic stimulation to be attained.

Entacapone is a selective, reversible COMT inhibitor. It does not cross the blood–brain barrier and acts primarily in the gut. Entacapone essentially increases both the peripheral and central availability of levodopa. The plasma elimination of a 200 mg oral dose of entacapone is 1–2 h. The pharmacokinetics of entacapone, particularly its elimination characteristics, are similar to those of levodopa, allowing coadministration of these agents. The recommended dose of entacapone is a 200 mg tablet administered with each dose of levodopa/carbidopa, up to a maximum of 10 times daily in Europe and 8 times daily in the United States. It should be noted that only the dose of levodopa should be titrated; the dose of entacapone administered with each dose of levodopa should remain the same, i.e. 200 mg.

Entacapone is effective in patients with wearing-off-type motor fluctuations and can produce an increase in "on" time and a reduction in "off" time by 60–90 min each per day. The most common adverse effect seen with entacapone is dyskinesia, which reflects increased central dopaminergic activity. Reducing the daily levodopa dosage by about 25% may be necessary to minimize possible dopaminergic adverse effects. This reduction may be made at the time of entacapone introduction in those patients on more than 800 mg of levodopa daily or in those with dyskinesias, but generally it is better to delay changing the levodopa dose until the patient's response can be evaluated. Physicians should be aware that dopaminergic adverse events generally occur within 24 h of initiating entacapone and may require an immediate adjustment of the levodopa dosage. Entacapone may be combined with both standard and controlled-release formulations of levodopa/carbidopa and may be administered with or without food.

The introduction in 2003 of Stalevo®, a combination of levodopa, carbidopa, and entacapone in one tablet, offered an opportunity to simplify the dosage regimen for patients on entacapone. Patients stable on levodopa and entacapone given separately can be converted directly to the equivalent dose of Stalevo. Stalevo tablets should not be cut or crushed; only one should be taken at each dose time and must not be combined with additional entacapone.

Tolcapone, unlike entacapone, can cross the blood–brain barrier and may produce some central COMT inhibition although the clinical effect of this action is likely to be minimal. A study in newly diagnosed, levodopa-naïve patients with PD failed to show any clinical efficacy with the introduction of tolcapone either alone or with selegiline. Tolcapone has a similar half-life to entacapone; however, owing to a greater bioavailability and smaller volume of distribution, tolcapone produces a greater inhibition of COMT and is only required on a t.i.d. regimen. Although tolcapone is available now both in Europe and North America, its use is restricted by its potential to cause severe hepatic toxicity. It should not be given to patients with impaired liver function, and those PD patients taking tolcapone require regular monitoring of hepatic enzymes. This toxic effect on liver function is not seen with entacapone and probably reflects their differing potency in inducing mitochondrial permeabilization. The use of tolcapone is generally limited to those patients who have failed to derive significant benefit from entacapone. Both entacapone and tolcapone can induce diarrhea, which is more common and may be severe and explosive with the latter.

3. Dopamine agonists

Several dopamine agonists are available for use in PD and fall broadly into two groups: ergot and non-ergot. Ergot agonists include bromocriptine, cabergoline, lisuride, and pergolide. Non-ergot agonists include apomorphine, piribedil, ropinirole, and pramipexole. Bromocriptine, cabergoline, pergolide, pramipexole, and ropinirole have all been studied for monotherapy use in early PD as well as for adjunctive treatment in more advanced PD. They have all demonstrated a significant beneficial effect on motor function and activities of daily living. Their side-effect profile is similar to levodopa in terms of inducing dopaminergic-related symptoms such as nausea, vomiting, and postural hypotension, but they are associated with a higher rate of peripheral edema, somnolence, and hallucinosis, particularly in the elderly. Somnolence with dopamine agonists is mainly seen during the early dose-escalation phase and patients should be warned of this and the rare but important side effect of sudden onset of sleep. In patients with early PD, mean age 61 years, hallucinosis also occurred more frequently during dose escalation but, like sedation, settles to a rate no higher than levodopa during maintenance.

The use of dopamine agonists is rarely associated with the development of pleural, pericardial, or peritoneal fibrosis. During the last 3 years reports have linked pergolide and cabergoline with fibrotic cardiac valvular disease in a pattern similar to that seen with other agents that also stimulate the $5HT_2$ receptor including methysergide and fenfluramine. There are insufficient data at present to know whether this complication is associated with ergot agonists alone, all dopamine agonists, or all dopaminergic drugs, and whether the effect is dose and/or time related.

Dopamine agonists and levodopa have been reported to cause behavioral abnormalities such as obsessive traits including compulsive shopping, gambling, and hypersexuality. These effects seem to be more common with dopamine agonists. Younger patients seem more susceptible, however (although older ones can be affected too), and these are the patients more likely to be on dopamine agonists. Thus, as with all dopaminergic-related side effects, caution is required before assuming that only one type of compound is causative.

Dopamine agonist monotherapy can effectively control dopaminergic symptoms for a period of time. Two follow-up studies of long-term monotherapy indicate that approximately 85%, 68%, 55%, 43%, and 34% of PD patients initiated on pramipexole or ropinirole are still controlled on monotherapy at 1, 2, 3, 4, and 5 years, respectively. This is dependent, however, upon the agonist being used at an appropriate dose. Nevertheless, patients will require levodopa supplementation at some point during their disease. If used correctly, it can produce symptom control comparable to levodopa. Although the studies cited above showed superiority for levodopa in UPDRS scores by up to five points, patients in the agonist arms had comparable quality-of-life scores and could have taken supplemental levodopa if the physician or patient felt it was required. The explanation for this discrepancy might be because the UPDRS does not capture all the benefit that a patient might derive from a dopamine agonist, including possible non-motor effects such as an antidepression action.

Several trials have now confirmed that bromocriptine, cabergoline, pergolide, pramipexole, and ropinirole are associated with a significantly reduced risk for the development of motor complications in comparison to levodopa (Fig. 2.4). In the pramipexole study, quality-of-life scores were also equivalent for the 4-year period. This implies that the patients were equally well controlled on agonist (with levodopa supplementation when required) or levodopa alone. Of course the levodopa group had more dyskinesias, but at 4 years these did not intrude significantly into patient quality of life, nor yet start to limit treatment options for motor control.

In conclusion, dopamine agonists provide effective control of PD-related motor symptoms with a good tolerance profile, delay the onset of motor complications, delay the introduction of levodopa, enable a lower dose of levodopa to be used, and in the case of pramipexole and ropinirole in particular, offer the possibility for some disease-modifying effect (see below).

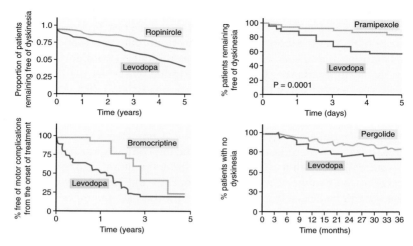

Figure 2.4 Dopamine agonists delay the development of dyskinesias. Results are from Rinne UK, Bracco F, Chouza C *et al.* Early treatment of Parkinson's disease with cabergoline delays the onset of motor complications. Results of a double-blind levodopa controlled trial. (The PKDS009 Study Group. *Drugs* 1998; 55(Suppl 1): 23–30; Rascol O, Brooks DJ, Korczyn AD, De Deyn PP, Clarke CE, Lang AE. A five-year study of the incidence of dyskinesia in patients with early Parkinson's disease who were treated with ropinirole or levodopa. 056 Study Group. *N Engl J Med* 2000; 342(20): 1484–91; and Parkinson Study Group. Pramipexole vs levodopa as initial treatment for Parkinson disease: A randomized controlled trial. *JAMA* 2000; 284(15): 1931–8.)

4. Monoamine oxidase B inhibitors

Two compounds of the propargylamine group, selegiline (deprenyl) and rasagiline, both of which are irreversible MAO-B inhibitors, have demonstrated symptomatic effect in PD patients and neuroprotective efficacy in the laboratory.

Selegiline has been available for several years and showed benefit as adjunctive treatment for PD. The DATATOP study was a prospective double-blind, placebo-controlled trial that investigated the effect of selegiline 5mg twice daily and/or 2000IU vitamin E as putative neuroprotective therapies. The time until PD patients required levodopa was used as the primary endpoint. No beneficial effect of vitamin E was detected at the dose given. In contrast, selegiline significantly delayed the need for levodopa compared to placebo, an effect consistent with slowing of disease progression. Selegiline was also found to exert a mild symptomatic effect, however, that confounded interpretation of the study. In a long-term follow-up study of the DATATOP cohort, levodopa patients who had been taking selegiline for 7 years compared to those who were changed to placebo after 5 years, had a significantly slower decline, less wearing-off, "on-off" and freezing, but more dyskinesias. Although one study did suggest that selegiline use might be associated with excess mortality, a recent large meta-analysis indicates that no such effect is evident and confirms the clinical efficacy of this drug in PD with total UPDRS score being improved by 2.7 points at 3 months. There is no evidence at present that MAO-B inhibition itself delays the development of motor fluctuations other than through the delay in introduction of levodopa and an ability to use a lower dose.

Rasagiline (*N*-propargyl-1(R)-aminoindan) is a relatively selective irreversible MAO-B inhibitor at recommended doses. This selectivity is important in avoiding the "cheese effect" of MAO-A inhibitors. Rasagiline is structurally related to selegiline, but is approximately 10 to 15 times more potent. It has good central nervous system penetration and a long half-life that allows a once-daily dosage schedule. Rasagiline is metabolized to aminoindan in contrast to selegiline which is metabolized to metamphetamine. This difference may have clinical relevance in terms of side-effect profile and the potential for disease modification (see below).

Rasagiline has been studied in patients with early PD. Patients were randomized to placebo or rasagiline (1 or 2 mg/day). In the placebo and rasagiline 1 mg and 2 mg groups, 81%, 83%, and 80%, respectively, were still on "monotherapy" at 6 months. There were no statistical differences in the rates for either levodopa supplementation or patient withdrawal. At the end of the 6-month period, the 1 mg rasagiline group had an improved UPDRS score compared to placebo of 4.2 units and 3.56 for the 2 mg group (Fig. 2.5). The degree of motor improvement over the 6-month period was comparable to that seen for selegiline in the DATATOP study, but not as great as that seen for dopamine agonists. There were no significant differences in the adverse-event profile between the treatment arms and placebo. At 6 months, the two treatment arms were almost back to their respective baseline UPDRS scores. The initial 6-month period was extended by a further 6 months. Patients were continued on their original dose of rasagiline or, if on placebo, were given rasagiline 2 mg/day. Patients requiring additional dopaminergic therapy were

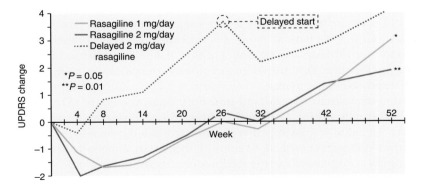

Figure 2.5 Twelve-month results of the TEMPO study: mean change in UPDRS-total. (From Parkinson Study Group. A controlled, randomized, delayed-start study of rasagiline in early Parkinson disease. *Arch Neurol* 2004; 61(4): 561–6.)

prescribed either levodopa or a dopamine agonist. For the whole 12-month period, deterioration from baseline scores was 3.01, 1.97, and 4.17 UPDRS units for the 1 mg, 2 mg, and delayed 2 mg cohorts. Those given rasagiline 1 mg/day for 12 months compared to those on the 2 mg dose for only the last 6 months maintained a total UPDRS improvement of 1.82 UPDRS units. The 12-month rasagiline 2 mg group had a 2.29-unit improvement over the 2 mg 6-month group. There was no significant excess of adverse events in the rasagiline arms compared to the placebo.

Two studies have been published on the efficacy of rasagiline in PD patients already taking levodopa. The PRESTO trial investigated PD patients on stable levodopa with at least 2.5 h of "off," i.e. poor motor state. Placebo decreased "off" time by 0.9 h (15% of "off" time) and rasagiline 1 mg/day by 1.9 h equating to 29% reduction of "off" time. Benefits were seen within 6 weeks of randomization and maintained throughout the 26-week study period. The improvement in "off" time was accompanied by a corresponding increase in "on" time, but 32% of the extra "on" time in the 1 mg group was with troublesome dyskinesia although this did not lead to any early terminations. The 1 mg rasagiline dose also resulted in significant improvements in the UPDRS score. The LARGO study investigated the effect of 1 mg/day rasagiline compared to entacapone or placebo in PD patients on stable levodopa but with at least 1 h of motor fluctuations per day. Placebo reduced "off" time by 0.4 h; both rasagiline and entacapone decreased "off" time by 1.2 h. There was a comparable and significant increase in "on" time without dyskinesias of 0.8 h with both drugs. These two studies demonstrate that once-a-day rasagiline (1 mg) significantly improves PD control in patients optimized on levodopa with or without additional therapy. Its efficacy is comparable to entacapone, but probably less than that of dopamine agonists which induce a 1- to 2-h improvement in PD control.

5. Other drugs

Anticholinergics were used to treat the symptoms of PD prior to the introduction of levodopa. Relatively little data are available on their potency and tolerance. Clinical trials have shown a modest benefit for anticholinergics in improving bradykinesia and rigidity, but this was at the expense of impaired cognitive function. Benztropine was equivalent to clozapine in producing a mild improvement in tremor.

Amantadine produces mild and transitory improvement in PD symptoms, benefits usually lasting 6–9 months, although some have suggested that the effects are more long lasting. It is generally considered unsuitable for monotherapy in PD and is mostly used as an adjunct. Improvements in bradykinesia and rigidity are generally of the same order of magnitude as anticholinergics, but their combination is additive. Amantadine use is also limited by its potential to induce cognitive defects.

II. Medical management

1. Initiation of treatment

Treatment for PD is always tailored to the specific needs and circumstances of the patient. Traditionally, drug treatment has only been initiated when the patient's symptoms interfere significantly with their employment or social activities. The rationale for this was very reasonable: the treatments available were considered symptomatic only, and incapable of modifying the course of the disease. Advances in our understanding of the pathophysiology and pharmacology of PD and the availability of new treatments for the disease have required us to reevaluate this strategy.

The clinical onset of PD motor features is directly associated with a series of functional changes in basal ganglia circuits and their target projections. Basal ganglia output becomes abnormal and clinical features appear when dopamine levels fall to <7% in 1-methyl-4-phenyl-1,2,3,6-tetrahydropyridine (MPTP)-treated non-human primates. The corresponding figure in humans is not known, but may be around 20–30%. The estimated asymptomatic latent period of approximately 6 years in idiopathic PD (and longer in familial PD) indicates the remarkable capacity of the basal ganglia to cope with progressively lower levels of dopamine, the compensatory mechanisms maintaining apparently normal motor function over the intervening years to diagnosis. These compensatory mechanisms include increased striatal dopamine turnover and receptor sensitivity, up-regulation of striatopallidal enkephalin levels, increased subthalamic excitation of the globus pallidus pars externa, and maintenance of cortical motor area activation. These observations, although neither completely defined nor understood, support the notion that declining dopamine levels during the early phase of PD put the basal ganglia level under stress. The onset of clinical symptoms denotes the point of failure to deal adequately with dopamine depletion. It might be that early correction of the basal ganglia functional abnormalities caused by dopaminergic cell loss and dopamine deficiency is a means to support the intrinsic physiological compensatory mechanisms and both limit and delay the circuitry changes that evolve as PD progresses. Review of the outcomes of the DATATOP, ELLDOPA, and TEMPO studies may support such a proposition. In these studies, those patients who received effective symptomatic treatment earlier in the course of their PD fared significantly better clinically than those initiated on placebo even when, as in the case of TEMPO, they were switched to the active drug after only 6 months.

Given the above, consideration of treatment initiation at the diagnosis of PD seems to be an increasingly viable and indeed attractive option for patients. Early restoration of basal ganglia physiology will support the compensatory events and delay the irreversible modification of circuitry that characterizes the clinical progression of PD. Such an effect may lead to lasting clinical benefit for the patient. Dopaminergic treatment can, however, be associated with unwanted side effects that may include gastrointestinal disturbances, cogni-

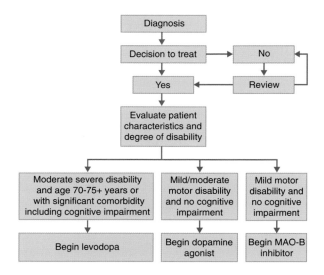

Figure 2.6 Decision pathway for the initiation of drug treatment for Parkinson's disease. (Schapira AH. *Arch Neurol* 2007; **64**(8): 1084. Copyright © 2007, American Medical Association. All rights reserved.)

tive problems, and sedation (see above). These need to be weighed against the symptomatic improvement that the patient will experience and the hypothetical long-term benefit outlined here.

Once an agreement has been reached between physician and patient on the introduction of drug therapy, consideration needs to be given to the choice of drug to start. As emphasized above, this needs to be individualized to the patient. The following, therefore, represents a general view of initiation options and is summarized in the algorithm of Fig. 2.6.

Those aged 75 years or younger with no cognitive impairment and no significant comorbidity should be considered for introduction of a dopamine agonist or an MAO-B inhibitor. The agonist will improve motor dysfunction more than an MAO-B inhibitor, but the latter is probably better tolerated. The choice between these agents will depend upon the patient's degree of symptomatic dysfunction. For those patients aged over 70 years, or those with cognitive dysfunction or significant comorbidity, levodopa would be the drug of choice for the initiation of therapy.

2. Maintenance of treatment (Fig. 2.7)

Most PD patients respond well to the initiation of dopaminergic therapy in small doses. Some require regular up-titration of their dose, however, before an adequate control of motor function is reached. This is particularly true of the dopamine agonists that may need to be increased (e.g. to 3 mg pramipexole

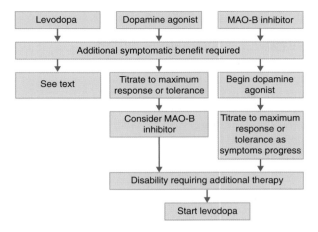

Figure 2.7 Decision pathway for the sequence and combination of drugs in early Parkinson's disease. (Schapira AH. *Arch Neurol* 2007; **64**(8): 1084. Copyright © 2007, American Medical Association. All rights reserved.)

or 12–15 mg ropinirole) before there is a good response. Some patients will need these doses to be increased yet further as their disease progresses. As indicated above, regardless of what drug is first used, PD patients will eventually require levodopa. This is most often introduced as a t.i.d. regimen, although the short half-life of the drug means that this falls well short of providing continuous dopaminergic stimulation. A higher frequency of administration would provide better symptom control and possibly less risk of the development of motor complications, but needs to be balanced against a probably lower rate of compliance.

3. Motor complications

The majority of PD patients will develop wearing-off or dyskinesias at some point in the course of their disease. Although the use of dopamine agonists will delay the onset, once levodopa is introduced the risk for their appearance increases. It is possible that the initiation of levodopa with a COMT inhibitor might delay the onset of motor complications, but evidence for this is lacking at present. The development of dyskinesias is probably related to dose of levodopa as well as duration and so the continuation of the dopamine agonist or MAO-B inhibitor to limit the levodopa dose is beneficial.

Wearing-off equates to the loss of effectiveness of a given dose of dopaminergic therapy and to the emergence of the primary motor features of PD (i.e. bradykinesia and rigidity) that still remain responsive to dopaminergic treatment. Patients recognize this as a return of symptoms prior to their next dose i.e. "end-of-dose failure," although some mistakenly associate it with the administration of the next dose given the medication's latency of effect. Wearing-off is eliminated by continuous administration of either levodopa or a dopamine agonist. While these methods are effective, they are not practical for the majority of patients. The simplest strategy is to increase the frequency of administration of levodopa, although this too may become difficult as dosage regimens increase to six or more times per day. Controlled-release formulations have proved disappointing with often little improvement in duration of response and problems with unpredictability of absorption and motor response. One open-label study demonstrated that the addition of cabergoline, a long-acting ergot dopamine agonist, to patients taking pramipexole or ropinirole, both non-ergots, resulted in improved motor control.

The addition of a COMT inhibitor to levodopa significantly improves "off" time (see above) and is an easy and effective strategy for managing wearing-off.

Dyskinesias are typically choreiform, occasionally dystonic involuntary movements induced predominantly by exposure to levodopa or other short-acting dopaminergic drugs. At first, the impact of dyskinesias on quality of life is limited. Patients may even be unaware of them, but they may be noticed by relatives or friends who are frequently more troubled by them than the patient. This changes, however, as dyskinesias become more severe. They not only cause difficulty and embarrassment to the patient, but also begin to restrict options for improving motor control.

The practical management of dyskinesias depends on the severity of the involuntary movements and their relationship to the medication dosage schedule. They may be peak dose, biphasic, or random. Peak-dose dyskinesias are related to high plasma concentrations of levodopa and can be managed by fractionating levodopa doses to avoid such peaks. This may or may not require an increase in the total daily dose. Alternative strategies include the introduction of a dopamine agonist if the patient is not already taking such an agent and if they remain a suitable candidate. Long-acting agonists are particularly useful in the management of dyskinesias, presumably owing to their ability to provide more continuous dopaminergic stimulation while avoiding rapid fluctuations in receptor stimulation. Biphasic dyskinesias occur when plasma levodopa concentration is rising or falling, and are associated with generally lower plasma levodopa concentrations. They tend to be more stereotypic and repetitive and to involve the lower extremities. They are more troublesome to manage but may respond to higher levodopa doses designed to keep the plasma concentrations above a critical level.

Amantadine has demonstrated efficacy in improving peak-dose dyskinesias. The effective dose is 200–400 mg per day in two divided doses, the severity of dyskinesias may be reduced by 24–56% and the effect sustained at 1 year.

The potential for the continuous parenteral administration of dopamine agonists or levodopa to improve or abolish motor fluctuations including dyskinesias has been discussed above. Apomorphine infusions or duodenal infusion of levodopa offer significant benefits for selected patients and can be considered an option prior to surgery (Fig. 2.8).

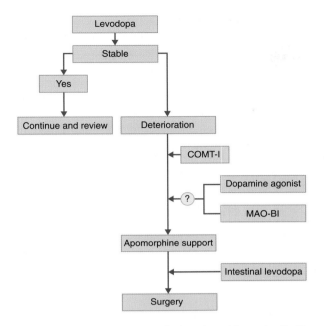

Figure 2.8 Decision pathway for the treatment of advancing and complex Parkinson's disease. (Schapira AH. Arch Neurol 2007;64(8):1084. Copyright © 2007, American Medical Association. All rights reserved.)

4. Management of non-motor complications

Depression and to some extent apathy (anhedonia) may respond to tricyclics such as amitriptyline, or to selective serotonin reuptake inhibitors (SSRIs). Pramipexole may be useful as an antidepressant, separate from its action to improve the motor features of PD. Anxiety and panic attacks can be prominent in PD and these may sometimes relate to wearing-off and so respond to strategies outlined above for this complication. Additional anxiolytic therapy may, however, be needed in some patients.

Hallucinations, if due to drugs, usually respond to a reduction in dose. In some patients, however, this is difficult owing to the re-emergence of motor features. Alternatively, hallucinations may respond to clozapine or quetiapine. Hallucinations are of course an important symptom of diffuse Lewy body disease, and their emergence early in the course of PD is a risk factor for dementia. PD patients who demonstrated dementia within 2 years of diagnosis showed a modest but significant improvement in cognitive function with rivastigmine, to a degree similar to that seen with this drug in Alzheimer's disease.

Several strategies are available to improve both nighttime sleep and daytime alertness in PD. These include improving sleep hygiene, treating nocturnal motor problems, better management of nocturia, modifying medication, and the use of modafinil in patients with refractory daytime drowsiness.

Viagra or apomorphine can in selected cases usefully manage the sexual dysfunction associated with PD. Bladder abnormalities particularly cause problems at night but can be improved by a range of options that include non-pharmacological as well as pharmacological strategies. The latter include the use of oxybutinin, tolterodine, or amitriptyline in patients with concomitant depression. Sialorrhea and drooling is often the result of reduced frequency of swallowing and may be helped simply by chewing gum or sucking sweets. Anticholinergic drugs may sometimes help, but often cause unwanted side effects. Botulinum toxin can be used for refractory cases.

Constipation and orthostatic hypotension are less common and are seen more often in the elderly population. Constipation usually responds to standard treatments, including increased fluid, bowel training, timing of evacuation to the patient being "on," and increased fiber intake. Symptomatic orthostatic hypotension may respond to simple advice regarding postural change, maintaining hydration, the use of pressure stockings, antidiuretic hormone, midodrine, or fludrocortisone.

III. Non-medical management

1. Surgery

Surgical approaches to the management of PD have been practiced since the mid-twentieth century. The discovery of dopamine depletion and the subsequent introduction of oral levodopa made surgery less attractive. The recognition of motor complications and the development of severe dyskinesias in some patients led to a resurgence of interest in lesioning the brain to control these features. Advances in surgical techniques, in neurophysiology and in molecular cell biology have provided the stimulus for the generation of a wide range of non-medical options for PD.

2. Destructive lesions

Thalamotomy may produce a reduction in tremor and bradykinesia. The best results have been achieved with lesion in the ventrointermediate (VIM) nucleus. Thalamotomy is not particularly helpful for bradykinesia or rigidity, however, and the procedure can be associated with significant morbidity related to the placement of the lesion. Thalamotomy has largely been replaced by medical therapies or deep brain stimulation (DBS).

Posteroventral pallidotomy can provide long-lasting improvement in contra-lateral dyskinesia and some improvement in bradykinesia and rigidity in PD patients. Like thalamotomy, pallidotomy has become less common as DBS has become more available. Both destructive lesions may still be offered, however, when symptoms significantly affect one side (bilateral destructive lesions cause increased complications including bulbar dysfunction) and when the opportunity for regular and expensive follow-up is limited.

Subthalamotomy has been shown to improve parkinsonian motor abnormalities including dyskinesias in animal models and in PD patients. Dyskinesia and hemiballismus have, however, also been reported following subthalamotomy, the latter being permanent in a few cases.

Deep brain stimulation was first proposed as a treatment in PD by Benabid based on his experience with high frequency stimulation as a means of confirming the target site for an ablative lesion. DBS can be used for bilateral procedures with relative safety. Also the stimulator can be adjusted to maximize benefits and reduce side effects. DBS simulates the effect of a destructive brain lesion but avoids the need to make such a lesion. The precise mechanism of action is unknown, but possibilities include depolarization blockade, release of inhibitory neurotransmitters, back firing, and/or inhibition of aberrant neuronal signals.

VIM DBS significantly improves contralateral tremor and is comparable in effect to destructive lesions but is superior in terms of side effects. Benefits are long-lasting, and have been shown to persist for more than 10 years. Only tremor is improved, however, and there is no effect on bradykinesia, rigidity, or dyskinesias. Thus VIM DBS is not as attractive as DBS of other targets. DBS of the subthalamic nucleus (STN) or globus pallidus pars interna (GPi) improve all of the cardinal features of PD as well as dyskinesias. Patients who could not be further improved with medical therapies (typically because of motor complications) experienced a substantial reduction in disability following DBS of the STN or GPi. Long-term studies demonstrate that benefits of DBS persist over more than 5 years of follow-up, although disability still progresses from year to year, reflecting degeneration in both dopaminergic and non-dopaminergic sites. There is now evidence from Deuschl and coworkers that DBS can improve quality of life more than optimized medical therapy in advanced disease.

Adverse events with DBS can be related to the intracranial procedure, the electrode system and stimulation. The surgical procedure can be associated with hemorrhage, tissue damage, and infection. In one multicenter study, 7 of 143 patients experienced hemorrhage, and neurological deficits persisted in four. Problems can also occur in relation to the device, including lead breaks, lead migration, infection and skin erosion. These occur in about 2–3% of cases and occasionally require replacement of the electrode. Severe depression and suicidal ideations or riotous laughing have been observed with stimulation of the STN, suggesting that basal ganglia circuits are involved with higher cortical and/or limbic as well as motor functions. The use of diathermy during surgical procedures should be avoided in patients with DBS as excess heat might be conducted to the brain by the electrode wire and cause necrosis.

DBS, particularly of the STN or GPi, now offers a significant benefit to those patients who suffer severe dyskinesias that are not controlled by standard means. Parkinsonian features are also improved, but no more than can be achieved by dopaminergic medication. DBS is relatively safe if performed by an experienced surgeon but still carries some small risk of permanent neurological deficit (often quoted as less than 1%). Patients should be carefully selected; those with cognitive impairment, acute psychiatric disease, or predominantly axial symptoms are excluded because of the risk of exacerbating this with surgery. Continuous follow-up is required and the procedure is expensive (see Chapter 3, case study 13).

3. Cell therapy

Fetal nigral transplantation has been evaluated in two double-blind, placebo-controlled studies. The first study randomized 40 patients to receive a transplantation or placebo procedure and followed them for 1 year. Modest benefits of transplantation were observed in UPDRS scores of activities of daily living and motor function in patients younger than 60 years of age. There was a significant increase in striatal fluorodopa uptake on positron emission tomography (PET), and there was modest survival of implanted cells at postmortem. The procedure was well tolerated, but approximately 15% of transplanted patients developed dyskinesias that persisted for days or weeks after levodopa was discontinued and were a source of major disability in some patients. Quality of life, the primary end point, was not improved. The second trial was a 2-year double-blind, placebo-controlled study that used a slightly different implantation protocol. Transplanted patients were not significantly improved in comparison to placebo patients, despite having significant increases in striatal fluorodopa uptake on PET and survival of implanted dopaminergic neurons at postmortem. Over half (56%) of the transplanted patients in this study developed dyskinesia during the practically defined "off" state when they had been held off levodopa for more than 12 h ("off-medication dyskinesia"). This phenomenon was not observed in non-transplanted patients. The precise mechanism responsible for off-medication dyskinesia remains unknown.

4. Growth factors

Glial-derived neurotrophic factor (GDNF) has attracted attention as a potential treatment for PD because of its capacity to protect or rescue dopaminergic neurons in tissue culture and in MPTP-treated monkeys. One open-label study used an infusion pump to directly administer GDNF into the striatum in five PD patients. There was an improvement in UPDRS motor scores during practically defined "off" periods as well as a small increase in striatal fluorodopa uptake around the catheter tip. A randomized controlled trial by Lang *et al.*, however, suggested that PD patients on GDNF were not significantly improved compared to placebo.

Gene and stem cell therapies are the subject of intense research but have yet to lead to clinically applicable treatments superior to those currently available.

IV. Neuroprotection

The limitations of symptomatic dopaminergic treatment has led to the search for agents to slow the progression of neurodegeneration in PD and thereby help prevent or slow clinical progression, or even reverse deficits by restoring normal function to defective neurons. It is accepted that such a strategy will only be successful if degeneration is ameliorated in multiple neurotransmitter systems, preventing the progression of both motor and non-motor features. The drugs that have received most attention in relation to neuroprotection include the MAO-B inhibitors and dopamine agonists, although others including coenzyme Q_{10}, growth factors, antiapoptotic agents, and glutamate inhibitors have also been the subjects of clinical trials in PD.

1. MAO-B inhibitors

Selegiline can protect cultured dopaminergic neurons against the toxicity of 1-methyl-4-phenylpyridinium (MPP^+) and in animal models can reduce dopaminergic cell loss in response to MPTP. Selegiline also protects against apoptotic cell death induced by serum and growth factor withdrawal, possibly via an increased production of Bcl-2. Selegiline, by virtue of its MAO-B activity, reduces the turnover of dopamine and thus free radical generation. The production of reactive oxygen species and free radical-mediated damage to lipids and proteins have been implicated in PD pathogenesis. These properties of MAO-B inhibition and reduced oxidative stress together with the ability of selegiline to protect against MPTP toxicity, led to the evaluation of this drug in the first clinical trial for neuroprotection in PD.

The results of the DATATOP study and others using selegiline and the TEMPO study investigating rasagiline have been discussed above. There seemed to be some benefit for selegiline, but interpretation is difficult in view of trial design and the compound's inherent symptomatic action. The results of the delayed-start design for TEMPO rasagiline were positive and support a neuroprotective action of the drug, but additional confirmatory trials are required before this drug can be accepted as neuroprotective.

2. Dopamine agonists

Dopamine agonists have antioxidant activity as a result of their hydroxylated benzyl ring structure. Numerous laboratory studies have demonstrated neuronal protection against free radical generating systems. These include attenuation of the effects of MPP^+, dopamine, 6-hydroxydopamine, and nitric oxide, and up-regulation of protective scavenging enzymes such as catalase and superoxide dismutase (SOD). These benefits are predominantly seen, however, at relatively high concentrations that may not be relevant in clinical practice. Dopamine agonists have demonstrated antiapoptotic activity in laboratory studies. For instance, pramipexole reduces cell death, prevents the release of cytochrome c and caspase activation in dopaminergic cells treated with MPP^+ or rotenone, and prevents a fall in mitochondrial membrane potential. Importantly, this dopamine agonist has also shown protective effects in the MPTP primate model of PD. Several studies suggest that dopamine agonists exert their protective effects not through stimulation of either D_2 or D_3 receptors, but rather via some alternative mechanism. The potential for dopamine agonists to protect non-dopaminergic cells, if translated to the clinic, would have pro-

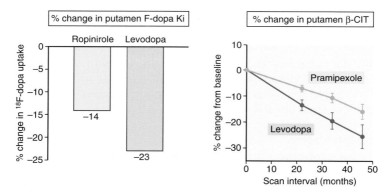

Figure 2.9 Results of SPECT and PET data from dopamine agonist neuroprotection studies. (From: Parkinson Study Group. Dopamine transporter brain imaging to assess the effects of pramipexole vs levodopa on Parkinson disease progression. *JAMA* 2002;287(13):1653-61; and Whone AL, Watts RL, Stoessl AJ *et al.* Slower progression of Parkinson's disease with ropinirole versus levodopa: The REAL-PET study. *Ann Neurol* 2003;54(1):93-101.)

found implications for disease modification and in particular for preventing the development of non-motor features in PD.

Two studies have sought to determine whether the neuroprotective benefits of dopamine agonists seen in the laboratory can be transferred to patients to modify the course of PD (Fig. 2.9). The CALM-PD study used 2β-carbomethoxy-3β-(4-iodophenyl)tropane (β-CIT) single photon emission computed tomography (SPECT) to follow the rate of loss of dopamine transporter as a marker of dopaminergic nigrostriatal cell density. Patients with early PD were randomized to pramipexole or levodopa and followed for a total of 4 years, levodopa supplementation was allowed in both arms. At 2, 3, and 4 years there was a significant reduction in the rate of transporter loss in the pramipexole group, averaging out at approximately 40%, consistent with the drug having a relatively protective effect in comparison to levodopa. A similar result was seen in the REAL-PET ropinirole study that used a similar trial design but used PET to follow loss of nigrostriatal cell density with fluorodopa. This demonstrated a circa 34% reduction over 2 years in the ropinirole group compared to those on levodopa. These studies have generated considerable interest and debate. Both studies demonstrate that dopamine agonists are associated with a significant delay in the rate of decline of a surrogate imaging marker of nigrostriatal function.

One interpretation of these findings is that these two dopamine agonists slow the rate of cell loss in the substantia nigra of PD patients, and this is consistent with the laboratory findings outlined above. Neither showed a corresponding clinical benefit, however, but it can be argued that the time course of the trials was too short to permit such an effect to be detected in the context of viable compensatory mechanisms and powerful symptomatic effects, and this will only become apparent with longer follow-up.

Another interpretation of these studies is that levodopa is toxic to nigral neurons. There is concern that levodopa might be toxic as it undergoes oxidative metabolism and has the potential to generate cytotoxic free radicals. Levodopa has been shown to be toxic to cultured dopamine neurons, but there is no convincing evidence that levodopa is toxic in *in vivo* models or in PD patients. The ELLDOPA trial investigated the possibility that levodopa may be toxic in PD patients but produced conflicting results. In this study, untreated PD patients were randomized to a total daily dose of 150, 300, or 600 mg of levodopa or placebo. β-CIT SPECT was used as an end point for integrity of the nigrostriatal system. Levodopa was associated with a significant increase in the rate of decline of imaging marker over 9 months compared to placebo, consistent with a toxic effect. Clinical evaluation, however, showed that those patients on levodopa had better UPDRS scores compared to placebo after 2 weeks of washout. This would, in contrast, be indicative of a protective effect of levodopa. Intellectual parsimony, however, would dictate that the simplest explanation for this clinical effect was that the washout period was too brief to eliminate the symptomatic benefits of levodopa.

Finally, it has been proposed that the differences between the effects of levodopa and dopamine agonists seen in the CALM-PD and REAL-PET studies are not related to any direct effect of the drugs on dopamine neuron survival or degeneration, but rather to a pharmacological difference in the capacity of these drugs to regulate the dopamine transporter or fluorodopa metabolism. A review of studies testing the effects of levodopa and dopamine agonists on transporter and fluorodopa metabolism, however, reveals that the data are conflicting and that at present there is insufficient information for or against such an effect.

In conclusion, the results of the two clinical trials of dopamine agonists using imaging end points support, but do not prove, a disease modifying effect in patients.

3. Coenzyme Q$_{10}$

Coenzyme Q$_{10}$ has been evaluated in a pilot study of early PD patients to determine whether it might have disease-modifying capabilities. The rationale for the use of coenzyme Q$_{10}$ in PD was based upon the observation that mitochondrial complex I activity is decreased in the PD substantia nigra, PD patients have reduced levels of coenzyme Q$_{10}$, and this compound protects against MPTP toxicity. Coenzyme Q$_{10}$ is both an antioxidant and an integral component of oxidative phosphorylation that has been shown to enhance electron transport. It is presumed not to have any symptomatic effect. Patients were randomized to either a placebo arm or one of three doses of coenzyme Q$_{10}$ (300 mg, 600 mg, or 1200 mg) and followed for 16 months. There was a significant benefit for coenzyme Q$_{10}$ 1200 mg in terms of change from baseline in total UPDRS compared to placebo at 16 months, and a non-significant trend to benefit for lower doses. This interesting and important result is sufficient to support further study of coenzyme Q_{10}, but insufficient at present to advocate that PD patients should use this compound.

4. Creatine

Creatine is converted to phosphocreatine and can transfer a phosphoryl group to adenosine diphosphate (ADP) to synthesize adenosine 5′-triphosphate (ATP) and so enhance energy production. It can reduce dopaminergic cell loss in the MPTP rodent model of PD. At a dose of 10 g daily, creatine was well tolerated and satisfied the predetermined criterion for non-futility based on time to requirement for symptomatic therapy for 66 early PD patients. Another blinded placebo-controlled study of 2 g daily for 6 months (after a loading dose of 20 g for 6 days) then 4 g daily for 18 months in 31 PD patients compared to 17 on placebo showed no significant difference in UPDRS scores or dopamine transporter density as assessed by SPECT. There was a significantly lower requirement for dopaminergic symptomatic treatment in the creatine arm, however, that could be indicative of a positive effect of creatine.

5. Antiapoptotic drugs

TCH346 is a drug that incorporates a propargyl ring within its molecular structure and so resembles selegiline. But since it does not inhibit MAO-B, it was not anticipated to have symptomatic effects in PD in clinical trials. TCH346 has been shown to prevent the death of dopamine neurons in various *in vitro* models of apoptosis, and to protect against behavioral abnormalities and neurodegeneration in animal models of PD. Propargylamines such as TCH346 have been shown to prevent the stress-induced translocation of glyceraldehyde-3-phosphate dehydrogenase (GAPDH) from the cytoplasm to the nucleus where it promotes nerve cell death by blocking the transcriptional up-regulation of protective molecules such as Bcl-2 and SOD. A trial of TCH346 in early untreated PD patients using three doses of the drug compared to placebo showed no benefit in the primary end point which was time to additional dopaminergic drug intervention. The reason for the failure to demonstrate effect may simply be due to TCH346 not acting as a neuroprotective agent in PD patients. Other possibilities, however, including use of an incorrect dose or a benefit that extended beyond the 12 to 18 months of the study cannot be excluded.

CEP1347 is a mixed lineage kinase inhibitor that should prevent apoptosis by intervening at the level of caspase activation. The results of the clinical trial of this drug have appeared only in abstract form, but have also failed to demonstrate clinical effectiveness.

V. Conclusion

The current range of medical and surgical therapies available for the treatment of PD is impressive. They offer excellent symptom relief for much of the duration of the disease. Their use is a complex matrix of decision-making that includes patient profile, disease stage, drug sequencing, and drug side effects. The use of surgical interventions, particularly DBS, has been an important advance for PD patients. Despite these important successes, there are two critical areas of unmet need; neuroprotection and adequate therapies for the non-motor features of PD. There is an important research focus on both these, however, and so new drugs and treatment strategies are likely to further improve the management of PD in the future.

Further reading

Barone P, Scarzella L, Marconi R *et al*. Depression/Parkinson Italian Study Group. Pramipexole versus sertraline in the treatment of depression in Parkinson's disease: a national multicenter parallel-group randomized study. *J Neurol* 2006; **253**(5): 601–7.

Chaudhuri KR, Healy DG, Schapira AH. Non-motor symptoms of Parkinson's disease: diagnosis and management. *Lancet Neurol* 2006; **5**: 235–45.

Deuschl G, Schade-Brittinger C, Krack P *et al*. German Parkinson Study Group, Neurostimulation Section. A randomized trial of deep-brain stimulation for Parkinson's disease. *N Engl J Med* 2006; **355**(9): 896–908.

Emre M, Aarsland D, Albanese A *et al*. Rivastigmine for dementia associated with Parkinson's disease. *N Engl J Med* 2004; **351**: 2509–18.

Fahn S, Oakes D, Shoulson I *et al*. Levodopa and the progression of Parkinson's disease. *N Engl J Med* 2004; **351**: 2498–508.

Goetz C, Koller W, Poewe W, Rascol O, Sampaio C. Management of Parkinson's disease: an evidence-based review. *Mov Disord* 2002; **17**(Suppl 4): S1–S166.

Goetz CG, Poewe W, Rascol O, Sampaio C. Evidence-based medical review update: pharmacological and surgical treatments of Parkinson's disease: 2001 to 2004. *Mov Disord* 2005; **20**(5): 523–39.

Holloway RG, Shoulson I, Fahn S *et al*. Pramipexole vs levodopa as initial treatment for Parkinson disease: a 4-year randomized controlled trial. *Arch Neurol* 2004; **61**: 1044–53.

Krack P, Batir A, Van Blercom N *et al*. Five-year follow-up of bilateral stimulation of the subthalamic nucleus in advanced Parkinson's disease. *N Engl J Med* 2003; **349**: 1925–34.

Lang AE, Lozano AM, Montgomery E, Duff J, Tasker R, Hutchinson W. Posteroventral medial pallidotomy in advanced Parkinson's disease. *N Engl J Med* 1997; **337**: 1036–42.

Limousin P, Krack P, Pollak P *et al*. Electrical stimulation of the subthalamic nucleus in advanced Parkinson's disease. *N Engl J Med* 1998; **339**: 1105–11.

Metman LV, Del Dotto P, LePoole K, Konitsiotis S, Fang J, Chase TN. Amantadine for levodopa-induced dyskinesias: a 1-year follow-up study. *Arch Neurol* 1999; **56**: 1383–6.

Nilsson D, Nyholm D, Aquilonius SH. Duodenal levodopa infusion in Parkinson's disease: long term experience. *Acta Neurologica Scand* 2001; **104**: 343–8.

Olanow CW, Obeso JA, Stocchi F. Drug insight: Continuous dopaminergic stimulation in the treatment of Parkinson's disease. *Nat Clin Pract Neurol* 2006; **2**(7): 382–92.

Pahwa R, Factor SA, Lyons KE *et al*. Quality Standards Subcommittee of the American Academy of Neurology. Practice Parameter: treatment of Parkinson disease with motor fluctuations and dyskinesia (an evidence-based review): report of the Quality Standards Subcommittee of the American Academy of Neurology. *Neurology* 2006; **66**(7): 983–95.

Parkinson Study Group. Effects of tocopherol and deprenyl on the progression of disability in early Parkinson's disease. *N Engl J Med* 1993; **328**: 176–83.

Parkinson Study Group. Pramipexole vs levodopa as initial treatment for Parkinson disease: A randomized controlled trial. Parkinson Study Group. *JAMA* 2000; **284**: 1931–8.

Parkinson Study Group. A controlled trial of rasagiline in early Parkinson disease: the TEMPO Study. *Arch Neurol* 2002; **59**(12): 1937–43.

Parkinson Study Group. Dopamine transporter brain imaging to assess the effects of pramipexole vs levodopa on Parkinson disease progression. *JAMA* 2002; **287**: 1653–61.

Parkinson Study Group. A controlled, randomized, delayed-start study of rasagiline in early Parkinson disease. *Arch Neurol* 2004; **61**: 561–6.

Parkinson Study Group. A randomized placebo-controlled trial of rasagiline in levodopa-treated patients with Parkinson disease and motor fluctuations: the PRESTO study. *Arch Neurol* 2005; **62**: 241–8.

Poewe W, Wenning GK. Apomorphine: an underutilized therapy for Parkinson's disease. *Mov Disord* 2000; **15**: 789–94.

Rascol O, Brooks DJ, Korczyn AD, De Deyn PP, Clarke CE, Lang AE. A five-year study of the incidence of dyskinesia in patients with early Parkinson's disease who were treated with ropinirole or levodopa. 056 Study Group. *N Engl J Med* 2000; **342**: 1484–91.

Rascol O, Brooks DJ, Melamed E *et al*. Rasagiline as an adjunct to levodopa in patients with Parkinson's disease and motor fluctuations (LARGO, Lasting effect in Adjunct therapy with Rasagiline Given Once daily, study): a randomised, double-blind, parallel-group trial. *Lancet* 2005; **365**: 947–54.

Schapira AH. Treatment options in the modern management of Parkinson disease. *Arch Neurol* 2007; 64: 1083–8.

Schapira AH, Bezard E, Brotchie J *et al*. Novel pharmacological targets for the treatment of Parkinson's disease. *Nat Rev Drug Discov* 2006; **5**: 845–54.

Schapira AH, Obeso J. Timing of treatment initiation in Parkinson's disease: A need for reappraisal? *Ann Neurol* 2006; **59**: 559–62.

Schapira AH, Olanow CW. Neuroprotection in Parkinson disease: mysteries, myths, and misconceptions. *JAMA* 2004; 291(3): 358–64.

Schrag A. Entacapone in the treatment of Parkinson's disease. *Lancet Neurol* 2005; **4**: 366–70.

Stacy M, Bowron A, Guttman M *et al*. Identification of motor and nonmotor wearing-off in Parkinson's disease: comparison of a patient questionnaire versus a clinician assessment. *Mov Disord* 2005; **20**: 726–33.

Van Camp G, Flamez A, Cosyns B *et al*. Treatment of Parkinson's disease with pergolide and relation to restrictive valvular heart disease. *Lancet* 2004; **363**(9416): 1179–83.

Whone AL, Watts RL, Stoessl AJ *et al*. Slower progression of Parkinson's disease with ropinirole versus levodopa: The REAL-PET study. *Ann Neurol* 2003; **54**: 93–101.

Yamamoto M, Uesugi T, Nakayama T. Dopamine agonists and cardiac valvulopathy in Parkinson disease: a case-control study. *Neurology* 2006; **67**: 1225–9.

Case study 1

Case presentation

A 67-year-old man was referred on January 2002 to the Sleep Disorders Clinic because of a 33-year history of talking, screaming, crying, laughing, punching, and kicking while asleep, as reported by his wife. Occasionally during these spells he had hit the bedside table or his wife, and had once fallen out of bed. The patient, unaware of this behavior, recalled having frequent nightmares such as being attacked or robbed. Rapid eye movement (REM) sleep behavior disorder (RBD) was considered.

The patient was a non-smoker. His previous medical history included arterial hypertension, and hyperlipidemia. One month prior to his visit to the Sleep Disorders Clinic, he had a right thalamic infarction during which he sustained transient sensory loss in his left-sided limbs. After this event he had been taking aspirin, enalapril, and simvastatin. Additionally, during the last year, he had been treated with sertraline 25 mg per day because of a 5-year history of depression. Treatment resulted in an improved mood. He had undergone surgery for removal of a benign prostatic hyperplasia 8 years before. About 2 years later, he developed erectile dysfunction and mild urinary urgency.

A one-night video-polysomnography in June 2002 revealed lack of atonia during REM sleep, associated with prominent limb jerking and talking, and confirmed the diagnosis of RBD. Brain magnetic resonance imaging (MRI) showed a right lacunar thalamic infarction but no other lesions. Sertraline was withdrawn without improvement of RBD symptoms. He was thought to suffer from idiopathic RBD and was started on clonazepam 0.5 mg at bedtime, with good response.

The patient described his sense of smell as having always been "poor" with no taste disturbances. There was no history of nose or head trauma, or sinusitis. He complained of troublesome constipation over the last 8 years, although he had never sought medical help for this.

The patient remained well over the next 3 years, during which sertraline was reintroduced because of a relapse of depression. In September 2005, at 71 years of age, right leg tremor appeared, spreading to his right upper limb within 1 month. The patient was referred then to the Movement Disorders Clinic where bradykinesia, rest tremor, and rigidity of the right arm and leg were detected. His face was slightly masked and his gait was normal, scoring 9 on Unified Parkinson's Disease Rating Scale (UPDRS) III. He was given a diagnosis of possible early Parkinson's disease (PD) (Hoehn & Yahr I; Schwab & England, 100%). A second brain MRI revealed no changes suggestive of other causes of parkinsonism. Dopamine transporter (DAT) single photon emission computed tomography (SPECT) showed bilateral decrease of striatal tracer uptake that was more pronounced on the left. Fourteen months later, in November 2006, parkinsonism had progressed (UPDRS-III score of 14; Hoehn & Yahr II), and the patient had modest functional impairment (Schwab & England, 90%). Pramipexole was introduced and gradually increased to 0.7 mg t.i.d., resulting in clinical improvement (UPDRS-III score of 6).

Differential diagnosis

Considering the diagnosis of probable early PD in the patient reported here, the presence of RBD [1,2], depression [3], constipation [4], and hyposmia [5,6] prior to the development of the cardinal motor symptoms can be seen retrospectively to be part of the neurodegenerative process and hence an example of premotor PD. Sertraline therapy could have been the cause of RBD (drug-induced RBD), but the persistence of symptoms after a prolonged drug washout period supported a diagnosis of idiopathic RBD. His mood disturbance resembled major depression, unrelated to PD. No information is available on whether premotor PD-related depression differs from primary depression in the essential clinical features and response to treatment. In light of the described link between depression and subsequent development of PD, it is now reasonable to consider that it may have been part of premotor PD in our patient. Other premotor features in this case, such as hyposmia or constipation, were mild and only documented when looked for through careful anamnesis.

A diagnosis of multiple system atrophy (MSA), a synucleinopathy in which progressive parkinsonism frequently occurs in association with dysautonomia and RBD, seems a possible alternative. RBD is very frequent in MSA and can also antedate the development of parkinsonism [2]. Urinary urgency and erectile dysfunction are also common in MSA and may antedate motor features in this disease as well. Several factors, however, do not favor the diagnosis of MSA in our patient. His asymmetrical, typical 4–6 Hz rest tremor and good response to dopaminergic treatment support PD. Furthermore, brain MRI lacked a putaminal hyperintense rim, characteristic of the parkinsonian variant of MSA. Although DAT SPECT is not helpful in distinguishing PD from MSA, the asymmetry in tracer uptake observed in this patient favors the diagnosis of PD. As for autonomic disturbances in this patient, both urinary urgency and erectile dysfunction were not progressive and were thought to be related to prostate surgery. This patient did not have symptomatic postural hypotension, which is very common in MSA and has been found to be more predictive of this synucleinopathy than urinary dysfunction. The presence of hyposmia, although not formally confirmed with smell tests, favors the diagnosis of PD as it is uncommon in atypical parkinsonisms including MSA [5].

Hence, the most likely diagnosis in this patient is PD. The symptoms of RBD, depression, hyposmia and constipation that antedated the classical motor features suggest that this neurodegenerative disorder might have started decades before the onset of motor symptoms.

Final diagnosis: PD with a history of premotor symptoms.

Discussion of premotor PD

Several studies have suggested that sleep disturbances (such as RBD), depression, constipation, and hyposmia, as well as other non-motor symptoms, can occur in the so-called premotor phase of PD [1–7]. These non-motor symptoms are thought to reflect involvement of non-dopaminergic structures in the central nervous system. Still, it is during this premotor phase that dopaminergic cell loss in the substantia nigra is thought to start, as has been suggested by neuroimaging studies [6,8]. DAT imaging of patients with unilateral PD, for example, has shown nigrostriatal dopamine loss contralateral to the clinically normal side.

RBD can precede the motor symptoms of PD by several years [1], and in one descriptive study, up to 20% of patients with RBD developed PD after a mean follow-up of 5 years [2]. Several studies have found that some PD premotor symptoms, such as hyposmia and impaired autonomic function (constipation, urinary, and bladder dysfunction), were more frequent in RBD patients than in controls, supporting RBD as a marker of underlying neurodegeneration and a premotor sign of PD [8,9].

Depression is common in PD and can occur in up to 27.6% of early PD patients. Depression has been shown to precede the development of motor manifestations in about 20% of cases [3]. It can predate PD diagnosis by as much as 20 years, but it occurs especially during the 3–6 years before the diagnosis. Depressed patients have a 2.24- to 3.22-fold risk for developing PD compared to non-depressed controls [3]. A recent study found a threefold rate of marked PD-like substantia nigra (SN) hyperechogenicity in depressed non-parkinsonian patients compared to the normal population [10].

Constipation and smell loss are other non-motor symptoms that are present frequently in *de novo* PD patients [4–7]. Epidemiological studies have shown that constipation can precede motor symptoms by many years [4]. The olfactory deficits are independent of disease severity and duration as they are detected even in untreated, newly diagnosed patients and are bilateral in patients with unilateral PD [5]. A case-control study found that 68% of PD patients reported hyposmia at the onset of motor deficits, whereas smell loss was only observed in 3% of controls [11]. In another study, 11 of 30 patients with idiopathic olfactory loss presented hyperechogenicity in the SN on transcranial sonography, five of whom featured decreased tracer uptake on DAT SPECT [6]. Olfactory dysfunction has also been observed in some asymptomatic relatives of patients with either familial or sporadic forms of PD, with some having altered DAT imaging [12]. In the Honolulu-Asia Aging Study, those who scored in the lowest tertile on the Brief Smell Identification Test were significantly more likely to have incidental Lewy body pathology [13]. Similar observations have been made in the same cohort regarding constipation [14]. Less well-studied premotor features of PD include anxiety, apathy, fatigue, non-specific pain, excessive daytime sleepiness, mid-life obesity, slow reaction time, and impaired color discrimination [7].

The recent proposal by Braak and coworkers that synuclein pathology (Lewy bodies and neurites) in PD progresses following a predictable caudal–rostral pattern lends support to the notion that some non-motor features can antedate the classical motor features of PD [15] (Table 3.1.1). Early hyposmia is in line with neuropathological changes observed in structures involved in the sense of smell, corresponding to the earliest neuropathological stage (stage 1). Similar clinicopathological correlations can be made regarding other premotor features such as constipation associated with degeneration of the dorsal nucleus of the vagus (stage 1), or even more peripherally and caudally at the level of the gastric and enteric plexuses. Premotor RBD can be linked to the early derangement of the pedunculopontine nucleus and the locus subcoeruleus (stage 2). The locus coeruleus and the raphe nuclei also in the mid brainstem have been implicated in the pathophysiology of depression in PD.

The study of the premotor phase of PD is of enormous importance as it could provide relevant information about where within the nervous system PD is beginning and what are its possible causes. However, this raises numerous challenges:
• How often and in what sequence do symptoms known to antedate the motor features of PD occur?
• What other symptoms should be looked for at this stage of disease development and in whom?

Table 3.1.1 Non-motor symptoms occurring in the premotor phase of PD

Symptoms	Potential CNS structures involved	Braak staging
Smell loss	Olfactory bulb, anterior olfactory nucleus	1
Depression	Locus coeruleus, raphe nuclei	2
Constipation	Dorsal nucleus of the vagus, enteric plexus neurons	1
REM sleep behavior disorder	Locus subcoeruleus, pedunculopontine nucleus	2

Other premotor manifestations of PD

Excessive daytime sleepiness, anxiety, pain, apathy and fatigue, mid-life obesity, impaired color discrimination

• Which neural structures are involved and what is the neuropathology of the premotor symptoms of PD: synuclein deposition, cell loss, neuronal dysfunction unrelated to α-synuclein deposition?

• How can individuals in the premotor phase of PD be identified? That is, when do symptoms like smell loss, RBD, or excessive daytime sleepiness represent premotor PD, and when do they not? Is imaging of the dopaminergic system with PET or SPECT useful in identifying such individuals?

• What is the risk of developing PD among individuals suffering from different combinations of these so-called premotor symptoms?

These and other questions remain unanswered today and are currently the focus of intense research. It is not possible now to reliably diagnose PD prior to the development of the cardinal motor signs. If treatment with disease modifying or neuroprotective potential in PD becomes available, identifying individuals in the premotor phase will become a serious priority. Application of such treatments in the premotor phase of PD could lead to a delay or prevention of the full-blown disorder.

Eduardo Tolosa, Carles Gaig, Yaroslau Compta, Alex Iranzo, Francesc Valldeoriola

References

1 Schenck CH, Bundlie SR, Mahowald MW. Delayed emergence of a parkinsonian disorder in 38% of 29 older men initially diagnosed with idiopathic rapid eye movement sleep behaviour disorder. *Neurology* 1996; **46**: 388–93.

2 Iranzo A, Molinuevo JL, Santamaría J *et al.* Rapid-eye-movement sleep behaviour disorder as an early marker for a neurodegenerative disorder: a descriptive study. *Lancet Neurol* 2006; **5**: 572–7.

3 Ishihara L, Brayne C. A systematic review of depression and mental illness preceding Parkinson's disease. *Acta Neurol Scand* 2006: **113**: 211–20.

4 Abbott RD, Petrovitch H, White LR *et al.* Frequency of bowel movements and the future risk of Parkinson's disease. *Neurology* 2001; **57**: 456–62.

5 Katzenschlager R, Lees AJ. Olfaction and Parkinson's syndromes: its role in differential diagnosis. *Curr Opin Neurol* 2004; **17**: 417–23.

6 Sommer U, Hummel T, Cormann K *et al.* Detection of presymptomatic Parkinson's disease: combining smell tests, transcranial sonography, and SPECT. *Mov Disord* 2004; **19**: 1196–202.

7 Tolosa E, Compta Y, Gaig C. The premotor phase of Parkinson's disease. *Parkinsonism Relat Disord* 2007; **13**(Suppl 1): S2–7.

8 Stiasny-Kolster K, Doerr Y, Möller JC *et al.* Combination of "idiopathic" REM sleep behaviour disorder and olfactory dysfunction as possible indicator for alfa-synucleinopathy demonstrated by dopamine transporter FP-CIT-SPECT. *Brain* 2005; **128**: 126–37.

9 Postuma RB, Lang AE, Massicotte-Marquez J, Montplaisir J. Potential early markers of Parkinson's disease in idiopathic REM sleep behavior disorder. *Neurology* 2006; **66**: 845–51.

10 Walter U, Hoeppner J, Prudente-Morrissey L, Horowski S, Herpertz SC, Benecke R. Parkinson's disease-like midbrain sonography abnormalities are frequent in depressive disorders. *Brain* 2007; **130**: 1799–807.

11 Henderson JM, Lu Y, Wang S, Cartwright H, Halliday GM. Olfactory deficits and sleep disturbances in Parkinson's disease: a case–control survey. *J Neurol Neurosurg Psychiatry* 2003; **74**: 956–8.

12 Ponsen MM, Stoffers D, Booij J *et al.* Idiopathic hyposmia as a premotoral sign of Parkinson's disease. *Ann Neurol* 2004; **56**: 173–81.

13 Ross GW, Abbott RD, Petrovitch H *et al.* Association of olfactory dysfunction with incidental Lewy bodies. *Mov Disord* 2006; **21**: 2062–7.

14 Abbott RD, Ross GW, Petrovitch H *et al.* Bowel movement frequency in late-life and incidental Lewy bodies. *Mov Disord* 2007; **22**: 1581–6.

15 Braak H, Del Tredici K, Rub U, de Vos RA, Jansen Steur EN, Braak E. Staging of brain pathology related to sporadic Parkinson's disease. *Neurobiol Aging* 2003; **24**: 197–211.

Case study 2

Case presentation

A 68-year-old professor of theology presented with a history of occasional involuntary tremulous movements affecting both hands and, to a lesser extent, the head. He described these rhythmical tremulous movements as only occurring when he was holding objects, for example when reading, drinking, or eating. At the time, he was being treated for depression with a selective serotonin reuptake inhibitor (citalopram 20 mg once daily) and he noted that in periods of anxiety, the tremulous movements were worse.

The patient maintained that both hands were affected symmetrically and that he had not observed this tremor when at rest with his hands supported by an armchair or when lying in bed. Furthermore, he had never noted tremor in the hands when standing with his arms hanging by his side.

His family history was unremarkable. He did not recall any of his relatives having suffered from tremor or other types of involuntary movements, and there were no known cases of Parkinson's disease (PD) in his family.

When the patient first consulted, both hands were affected by a clear postural and action tremor with mild amplitude and a frequency of approximately 8–10 Hz. Subtle asymmetry was noticeable with slightly larger tremor amplitudes in the left hand, but no rest tremor. There was no detectable rigidity in his arms or legs, and no slowing of speed or amplitude of rapid finger or hand movements. His gait and arm swing were normal. His facial expression was somewhat diminished and he spoke with a low and soft voice. He acknowledged feeling depressed.

The patient was given a diagnosis of possible essential tremor. He was told that there was no clinical sign of his tremor being caused by PD, but that there was a possibility that citalopram might be a contributor. He was given a prescription for propranolol with a starting dose of 10 mg twice daily to be increased in 10-mg increments to 2 × 20 mg if needed.

When seen again approximately 12 months later, the patient reported that he had decided not to take propranolol. His family physician had recommended biperiden instead, but he had likewise refrained from taking this drug. He felt that the tremulous movements had become worse and would now sometimes appear at rest, such as when sitting quietly watching TV. He felt no reduction in his overall mobility, and no loss of dexterity in his hands other than the tremor. He described his walking as normal and his depression as slightly improved.

At the time of this examination, the patient again displayed roughly symmetrical postural and kinetic tremor affecting both hands. During the examination there were two very brief episodes where a right-sided resting tremor became apparent. There was still no sign of rigidity in his extremities or at the neck, no slowness or amplitude reductions in repetitive movements of his fingers or hands, and gait was still normal.

A dopamine transporter (DAT) single photon emission computed tomography (SPECT) imaging study was ordered and revealed a disturbance of the presynaptic DAT system on both sides of the striatum (ratio between striatum and cerebellum: right, 3.2; left, 3.4). A levodopa test was performed and continuous treatment with levodopa was started. Since then, the patient has been on regular oral levodopa (100 mg t.i.d.) with overall acceptable tremor control, but he still describes tremor breakthroughs in emotionally tense situations. His overall mobility has not been affected. He still plays the piano and he goes for long walks without difficulty. Recently, he had dystonic cramps in the toes of the right foot.

Discussion

On his first consultation, the patient fulfilled the Movement Disorder Society consensus criteria for the diagnosis of essential tremor (ET) [1], presenting with a mild postural and action tremor affecting both hands, with a frequency of approximately 8–10 Hz and without PD features or other neurological signs.

Interestingly, after 12 months a parkinsonian tremor became apparent, presenting as unilateral resting tremor with a frequency of 4–6 Hz [1]. The parkinsonian tremor occurred in the right arm and showed a good response to levodopa. There was still no detectable rigidity in his arms or legs and no slowing of speed or amplitude of rapid finger or hand movements.

This case is instructive for a number of reasons, as given below.

Do ET patients carry a higher risk for developing PD than normal controls? ET is the most common adult movement disorder with a prevalence ranging from 2.8% to 4% in individuals aged over 40 years, and a prevalence of 14% in people older than 65 [2]. The prevalence of PD is estimated at 1.6% [3]. The incidence of both ET and PD increases with age, and coexistence of these frequent movement disorders in a single patient may occur by chance, but several studies have reported an association between ET and PD [4]. Some studies have found that ET patients carry an increased risk for PD compared with the general population, and studies have described an increased risk for PD in first-degree relatives of ET patients [5]. One study showed that 70% of twins with postural tremor had PD themselves or a twin with PD [6]. In a study of 678 ET patients, of whom 6.1% had PD features, the authors concluded that the frequency of PD in ET is more than that reported in the general population [7].

A further link between a subset of ET patients and PD is supported by pathological findings in the brains of ET patients. Six out of ten ET patients studied at the Essential Tremor Centralized Brain Repository at Columbia University exhibited a distinctive pattern of Lewy bodies in the locus coeruleus. This observation further supports the theory that a proportion of ET patients could have a form of Lewy body disease [8]. All these studies lead to the hypothesis that our patient, who subsequently developed a parkinsonian tremor, may reflect a subgroup of ET patients at higher risk for developing PD.

The concept of "benign tremulous PD." In our patient, tremor remains the predominant feature in the course of the disease. Hypokinetic symptoms are still mild and do not seem to progress, despite a disease duration of 8 years. Several studies have examined possible risk factors for the progression of PD. Roos *et al.* showed that patients with tremor reach Hoehn & Yahr (HY) stage III significantly later than patients with hypokinesia and rigidity [9]. Marttila & Rinne found that patients presenting predominantly with tremor had a better prognosis than those presenting with other parkinsonian signs [10]. Of those patients starting with tremor, 70% remained in HY stage I and II, compared to 60% of those starting with other symptoms.

Recently, a study of 16 PD patients with tremor as the predominant feature and only mild progression called this condition "benign tremulous parkinsonism" or "isolated tremor with very mild parkinsonian signs" [11]. The authors concluded that benign tremulous parkinsonism may be a distinct entity characterized by tremor predominance (often not very responsive to levodopa therapy) with minimal progression of other aspects of parkinsonism. The clinical presentation of this form of parkinsonism reflects the heterogenicity of neurodegenerative diseases. Whether patients with tremor as the predominant feature and mild progression exhibit a different pathophysiology will have to be elucidated in further studies.

DAT-SPECT investigation into the differential diagnosis of parkinsonian and non-parkinsonian tremor. Despite different phenomenology, the differentiation of parkinsonian and non-parkinsonian tremor may be a diagnostic challenge. There may also be some doubt in differentiating between "true" rest tremor and incomplete muscle relaxation in patients with moderate postural tremor.

The use of DAT SPECT has been shown to facilitate the differential diagnosis in patients with isolated tremor symptoms [12]. Loss of function of the striatal dopamine nerve terminal is a hallmark of neurodegenerative parkinsonism and is strongly related to a decrease in DAT density. This can be measured by SPECT. Patients with possible ET without other neurological features consistently have normal DAT imaging. Some SPECT studies are thought to be 90% sensitive in differentiating PD from normal subjects or ET. Brooks *et al.* [13] showed that patients with isolated rest tremor had consistently abnormal striatal ^{18}F-dopa uptake, whereas those with isolated postural tremor did not. Lee *et al.* performed a brain SPECT study in patients with a long duration of isolated postural tremor, in whom rest tremor developed after the onset of postural tremor [14]. Many of these patients demonstrated reduced levels of striatal DAT, comparable to levels seen in typical PD. The authors concluded that later in their clinical course, some patients with postural tremor may acquire rest tremor in association with mild substantia nigra neuronal loss. Chaudhuri *et al.* showed that long-standing isolated asymmetrical postural tremor may evolve to PD, supported in 5 of 13 reported cases (38%) by abnormal [123I] 2β-carbomethoxy-3β-(4-iodophenyl)tropane (β-CIT) SPECT, whereas uncertain parkinsonian signs and normal [123I]FP-CIT led to a change of diagnosis to ET in 5 of 24 cases [15].

In our patient, DAT SPECT imaging revealed a disturbance of the presynaptic DAT system on both sides of the striatum. These results provided helpful additional information, leading to the diagnosis of early PD and the initiation of levodopa therapy. DAT SPECT imaging may differentiate parkinsonian tremor from essential tremor and confirm the diagnosis of early PD in ET patients who subsequently develop parkinsonian tremor with only subtle extrapyramidal signs.

Final diagnosis: early Parkinson's disease.

Heike Stockner, Werner Poewe

References

1 Deuschl G, Bain P, Brin M. Consensus statement of the Movement Disorder Society on Tremor. Ad Hoc Scientific Committee. *Mov Disord* 1998; **13**(Suppl 3): 2–23.

2 Wenning GK, Kiechl S, Seppi K *et al.* Prevalence of movement disorders in men and women aged 50–89 years (Bruneck Study cohort): a population-based study. *Lancet Neurol* 2005; **4**: 815–20.

3 De Rijk MC, Tzourio C, Breteler MM *et al.* Prevalence of parkinsonism and Parkinson's disease in Europe: the EUROPARKINSON Collaborative Study. European Community Concerted Action on the Epidemiology of Parkinson's disease. *J Neurol Neurosurg Psychiatry* 1997; **62**: 10–15.

4 Shahed J, Jankovic J. Exploring the relationship between essential tremor and Parkinson's disease. *Parkinsonism Relat Disord* 2007; **13**(2): 67–76.

5 Jankovic J, Beach J, Schwartz K, Contant C. Tremor and longevity in relatives of patients with Parkinson's disease, essential tremor, and control subjects. *Neurology* 1995; **45**: 645–8.

6 Tanner CM, Goldman SM, Lyons KE *et al.* Essential tremor in twins: an assessment of genetic vs environmental determinants of etiology. *Neurology* 2001; **57**: 1389–91.

7 Koller WC, Busenbark K, Miner K. The relationship of essential tremor to other movement disorders: report on 678 patients. Essential Tremor Study Group. *Ann Neurol* 1994; **35**: 717–23.

8 Louis ED, Vonsattel JP, Hong LS, Ross GW, Lyons KE, Pahwa R. Essential tremor pathology: a case-control study from the essential tremor centralized brain repository. *Mov Disord* 2005; **20**: 1241.

9 Roos RA, Jongen JC, van der Velde EA. Clinical course of patients with idiopathic Parkinson's disease. *Mov Disord* 1996; **11**(3): 236–42.

10 Marttila RJ, Rinne UK. Progression and survival in Parkinson's disease. *Acta Neurol Scand Suppl* 1991; **136**: 24–8.

11 Josephs KA, Matsumoto JY, Ahlskog JE. Benign tremulous parkinsonism. *Arch Neurol* 2006; **63**: 354–7.

12 Scherfler C, Schwarz J, Antonini A *et al*. Role of DAT-SPECT in the diagnostic work up of Parkinsonism. *Mov Disord* 2007; **22**(9): 1229–38.

13 Brooks DJ, Playford ED, Ibanez V *et al*. Isolated tremor and disruption of the nigrostriatal dopaminergic system: an 18F-dopa PET study. *Neurology* 1992; **42**: 1554–60.

14 Lee MS, Kim YD, Im JH, Kim HJ, Rinne JO, Bhatia KP. ^{123}I-IPT brain SPECT study in essential tremor and Parkinson's disease. *Neurology* 1999; **52**(7): 1422–6.

15 Chaudhuri KR, Buxton-Thomas M, Dhawan V, Peng R, Meilak C, Brooks DJ. Long duration asymmetrical postural tremor is likely to predict development of Parkinson's disease and not essential tremor: clinical follow up study of 13 cases. *J Neurol Neurosurg Psychiatry* 2005; **76**(1): 115–17.

Case study 3

Case presentation

A 32-year-old man with no history of neurological disease presented with gait disorder and tremor. First symptoms appeared 6 months ago with gradual progression. For the past year, he had been tired with difficulties concentrating, especially at work. Friends and family members had noticed behavior modifications, with inappropriate joviality or irritability. His gait was unsteady, cautious and with small steps. Arm swing was reduced. On examination, bilateral extrapyramidal rigidity and akinesia of the upper limbs was observed, with slight axial rigidity. There was no rest tremor, but a postural tremor when the patient's arms were outstretched. In view of his fatigue, his primary care physician had prescribed a blood test that revealed a thrombocytopenia (platelets, 60 000/mm^3). Liver tests were normal. Biological examinations guided us to the diagnosis.

Differential diagnosis

Idiopathic Parkinson's disease (PD): The clinical presentation of this patient indicates a parkinsonian syndrome, with akinesia and extrapyramidal rigidity. However, the initial absence of asymmetry, the nature of the tremor and his biological anomalies make it necessary to continue our investigation before settling on a diagnosis of idiopathic PD.

Genetic PD: When a parkinsonian syndrome is encountered in such a young patient, a genetic cause must be considered. With a mutation of the *Parkin* gene, the disease generally starts earlier. The patient's thrombopenia, action tremor without rest features, and his behavioral problems, however, do not concur with this hypothesis.

Wilson's disease (WD): The association of behavioral abnormalities, parkinsonian syndrome and action tremor is highly suggestive of WD. The absence of any abnormalities in the liver tests does not rule out the hypothesis of WD, especially in its neurological forms.

Table 3.3.1 Biological results

	Value	Normal range
Ceruloplasmin	0.1 g/L	0.22–0.61
Serum copper	4.51 µmol/L	12.7–22.2
Urinary copper	2.45µmol/24h	0.2–1.0

The diagnosis of WD is suggested by a decrease in serum copper and ceruloplasmin levels and an increase in 24-h urinary copper excretion (Table 3.3.1). Serum copper level is less helpful, as it reflects total copper levels and not free toxic copper (i.e. non-ceruloplasmin-bound). Slit-lamp examination revealed a Kayser–Fleischer (K-F) ring (Fig. 3.3.1). Fluid-attenuated inversion recovery (FLAIR) magnetic resonance imaging (MRI) revealed hypersignals in the central gray matter and in the cerebellar peduncles (Fig. 3.3.2). These explorations (biological, ocular, and MRI) enabled the diagnosis to be confirmed and treatment to be initiated, even before receiving the results of the direct

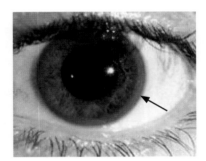

Figure 3.3.1 Kayser–Fleischer ring.

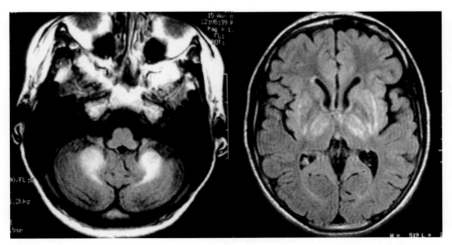

Figure 3.3.2 FLAIR MRI with hypersignals in the central gray matter and in the cerebellar peduncles.

genetic analysis. This analysis found one H1069Q mutation of the *ATP7B* gene on chromosome 13 (exon 14). Even though a second mutation was not found (autosomal recessive disorder), this does not rule out the diagnosis.

Final diagnosis: Wilson's disease.

Discussion

Wilson's disease is an autosomal recessive disorder linked to a mutation of the *ATP7B* gene mapped to chromosome 13. The ATP7B protein plays an essential role in copper homeostasis (Fig. 3.3.3). Its two main functions are first to bind copper to ceruloplasmin to avoid toxic unbound copper from circulating in the blood, and second to transport excess hepatic copper into the bile canaliculus for excretion, thereby preventing copper overload [1].

Diagnosis of WD can be made at various stages in the illness: (1) the pre-symptomatic stage following family testing or the fortuitous discovery of biological anomalies; (2) the hepatic stage with liver failure, cirrhosis or fulminant hepatitis; and (3) the neurological stage [2]. The hepatic form is more common in children. The neurological form occurs in young adults, but some rare cases have been observed later (up to 55 years of age in our personal cohort).

There are three main neurological manifestations:

• Dystonic syndrome starts with focal signs or with functional dystonia and, if left untreated, progresses to generalized dystonia. It often affects facial muscles, resulting in a fixed sardonic smile. A dystonic dysarthria can touch laryngeal or pneumophonatory muscles and may be associated with choreic movements.

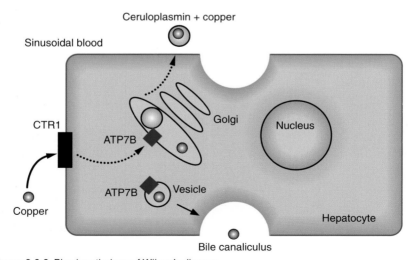

Figure 3.3.3 Physiopathology of Wilson's disease.

• Parkinsonian syndrome causes rigidity and akinesia, as seen in our patient. Hypomimia is present, as well as dysarthria with hypophonia, tachylalia, and sometimes pseudo stuttering. Gait is unsteady with small steps, reduced postural reflexes with instability on turning around, reduction in arm swing, festination, and freezing. Rest tremor is rarely isolated.

• The trembling form is characterized by postural and action tremor with high amplitude and low frequency, and increases with goal-directed movement. Its proximal component can be well observed when a patient's arms are outstretched in what is called wing-beating tremor. This tremor can also be associated with cerebellar syndrome.

These neurological manifestations often occur simultaneously as illustrated by the patient presented here [3].

On a neuropsychological level, patients often suffer from a dysexecutive syndrome linked to subcorticofrontal lesions. Attention deficits can cause difficulties in professional activities. Psychiatric disturbances can be limited to behavioral changes or irritability. Depression is frequent. Psychotic disturbances are rare, but can sometimes be the starting point of the illness.

The initial biological exploration should include serum copper levels (low or normal), serum ceruloplasmin levels (low in 90% of cases) and 24-h urinary copper excretion (increased). In our experience, a K-F ring (a deposition of copper at the periphery of the cornea) is always present in the neurological form of the disease (>98% in the literature [1]). Structural brain MRI is always abnormal, revealing widespread atrophy and hypersignals in FLAIR and diffusion sequence in the basal ganglia, cerebellar peduncles, and the mesencephalus [4]. Hyposignals in FLAIR and T2 sequences can be seen at a later stage of the illness. In hepatic forms with a portacaval shunt, bilateral hypersignals in the striatum can be seen on T1 sequences, although these are not specific to WD.

Liver exploration results can be normal in neurological forms of the disease, even if the liver is histologically overloaded with copper or there is cirrhosis with hypersplenism, which explains our patient's thrombopenia. A biopsy is not necessary for the diagnosis in the majority of neurological forms. It can, however, be useful for the diagnosis and prognosis in hepatic forms to weigh intrahepatic copper and to evaluate the degree of fibrosis.

On a genetic level, we now know of more than 350 mutations of the "Wilson" gene. There is no genotype–phenotype correlation and the discovery of a mutation does not automatically enable the prognosis or the response to treatment to be determined. As in this case, the two mutations cannot always be found. Family testing, based on indirect genetic analysis (haplotype study) is important to detect presymptomatic forms among siblings early and to treat these before symptoms appear. Our patient had a heterozygous brother – an unaffected carrier who can transmit the gene.

Once the diagnosis of WD is confirmed, it is necessary to give life-long treatment. Treatment options are the copper chelators D-penicillamine and triethylene tetramine (TETA), and zinc salts.

• D-penicillamine is the treatment of choice for symptomatic forms of WD and its efficacy has been well established. Its use, however, requires regular clinical and biological monitoring owing to numerous side effects. Early side effects include immunoallergic reactions or glomerulopathy, while lupus and elastopathy have been observed later. Our patient was given increasing doses of D-penicillamine to reach a daily dose of 1500 mg.
• TETA has fewer side effects than D-penicillamine. It is used either as initial treatment for symptomatic Wilson's disease, or as replacement therapy if D-penicillamine is poorly tolerated.
• Zinc salts reduce digestive copper absorption. This treatment is well tolerated with few digestive side effects. This is the first-line treatment for pre-symptomatic forms of the disease. It is also prescribed as maintenance therapy to replace initial chelator treatment once the disease has been stabilized. In severe forms, a chelator and zinc can be combined.

Neurological worsening is more frequent with D-penicillamine (14%) than with TETA (8%) or zinc (4%) [5].

Ammonium tetrathiomolybdate is a promising drug especially in early stages of the disease, but needs further study to determine how it can be best used in disease management.

Liver transplant is necessary in cases of acute hepatitis, but is open to discussion when neurological deterioration continues despite treatment.

In our patient, neurological symptoms improved after 6 months of treatment. After 2 years, his gait was normal and trembling, slight. He, nevertheless, continued to have behavioral abnormalities.

Response to treatment varies from patient to patient. Among those studied by Merle *et al.* [6], 54% of patients with neurological symptoms improved with treatment, 22% showed a stable neurological condition and 24% experienced worsening of symptoms. These data highlight the need to diagnose the disease as early as possible and the importance of family screening to treat patients before symptoms appear.

Jean-Marc Trocello, France Woimant

References

1 Ala A, Walker AP, Ashkan K, Dooley JS, Schilsky ML. Wilson's disease. *Lancet* 2007; **369**: 397–408.
2 Woimant F, Chaine P, Favrole P, Mikol J, Chappuis P. La maladie de Wilson. *Rev Neurol (Paris)* 2006; **162**: 6–7, 773–81.
3 Machado A, Chien H, Deguti M *et al.* Neurological manifestations in Wilson's disease: report of 119 cases. *Mov Disord* 2006; **21**(12): 2192–6.
4 Favrole P, Chabriat P, Guichard JP, Woimant F. Clinical correlates of cerebral water diffusion in Wilson's disease. *Neurology* 2006; **66**: 384–9.
5 Ferenci P, Członkowska A, Merle U *et al.* Late-onset Wilson's disease. *Gastroenterology* 2007; **132**: 1294–8.
6 Merle U, Schaefer M, Ferenci P, Stremmel W. Clinical presentation, diagnosis and long-term outcome of Wilson's disease: a cohort study. *Gut* 2007; **56**: 115–20.

Case study 4

Case presentation

A 47-year-old man initially presented an asymmetrical resting tremor in the right leg and soon after, in the left leg as well. He was diagnosed with Parkinson's disease (PD) and treated with levodopa which improved his symptoms by 80% according to his own estimation. When the patient was first examined by us 14 years after the onset of the disease, he was 61 years old and presented the typical parkinsonian triad with bradykinesia, rigidity, and resting tremor. Levodopa responsiveness remained marked and improvement reached 70% with treatment. He fulfilled the diagnostic criteria for definite PD and presented no atypical signs – extensor plantar response, ophthalmoplegia, dementia (MMS was 30/30), or autonomic failure. His Unified Parkinson's Disease Rating Scale (UPDRS) score 3 h after 150 mg of levodopa and 2.5 mg of bromocriptine was 31, and his Hoehn & Yahr score, 2.5. Cerebral magnetic resonance imaging (MRI) was normal.

There was a positive family history of parkinsonism. His father, who had died at the age of 75, apparently had parkinsonism. His brother presented extrapyramidal symptoms, but they were attributed to antipsychotic therapy prescribed for bipolar disorder. Our patient had never taken neuroleptic drugs.

Twenty-three years after the onset of symptoms, the patient presented severe gait instability. Neurological examination at this time showed predominant parkinsonism but also pyramidal signs (brisk reflexes in upper and lower limbs, bilateral Babinski sign) and loss of vibration sense in his lower limbs. Ocular pursuit was saccadic without ophthalmoplegia. There was also cognitive impairment with a Mini Mental State Examination score of 22/30. The response to levodopa persisted, and interruption of treatment induced severe motor degradation. Electrophysiological data confirmed the existence of sensory and motor axonal neuropathy. Cerebral MRI showed only moderate cerebellar atrophy involving both the vermis and the hemispheres.

Differential diagnosis

Genetic molecular analyses were proposed on the basis of our patient's family history and the early onset of his parkinsonism which was too early for idiopathic PD. Wilson's disease with autosomal recessive inheritance was not investigated because onset was too late and the family history was consistent with dominant transmission. Among autosomal dominant PD genes, the common G2019S mutation in the *LRRK2* gene was excluded. As the final neurological examination suggested a more diffuse neurodegenerative disorder with pyramidal and cerebellar involvement, supported by MRI findings, analysis of the *SCA2, 3* and *17* genes was proposed. No expansions were detected at the SCA3 and SCA17 loci, but we found an expanded SCA2 allele with 37 CAG repeats.

Final diagnosis: spinocerebellar ataxia.

Discussion

Spinocerebellar ataxias (SCAs) are a heterogeneous group of autosomal dominantly inherited, progressive neurodegenerative diseases linked to more than 28 loci. These diseases are often caused by expansion of trinucleotide repeats encoding polyglutamine (polyQ) tracts. Although ataxia is often the predominant symptom, the phenotype and the age at onset are highly variable, even within families. Extrapyramidal features consistent with neuropathological evidence of basal ganglia involvement may also occur [1]. Parkinsonism has been reported in *SCA1, 2, 3, 7* and *17*. *SCA2* is the second most frequent SCA gene worldwide and is linked to expansion of a CAG nucleotide repeat in the coding region of the ataxin-2 gene, located on chromosome 12q23–24. Most normal alleles range from 14 to 31 repeats, whereas the expanded alleles have from between 34 and 35 to approximately 200 repeats.

SCA2 expansion results in typical PD. Expansion of *SCA2* CAG repeats usually results in progressive cerebellar gait and limb ataxia, dysarthria with slow saccades, and decreased tendon reflexes. The phenotype, however, is almost always enriched by the variable association of pyramidal and extrapyramidal signs, peripheral neuropathy, cognitive signs, and other ophthalmologic features. This clinical variability is partly accounted for by the size of the expansion [2]. Our patient presented typical levodopa-responsive parkinsonism, with no additional neurological features at least until his last examination. As previously reported, *SCA2* has been recognized as an uncommon cause of pure parkinsonism, indistinguishable from idiopathic PD [3–10].

SCA2 expansions mimicking PD are rare in families with autosomal dominant parkinsonism (ADP). In our series of patients with familial PD, *SCA2* expansions were detected in 3 of 164 ADP families, which represents 2% [10]. This result is consistent with previous studies where *SCA2* expansions contributed to familial parkinsonism with variable frequencies according to ethnic origin (Table 3.4.1). The range in Caucasians was 0–2% [4,7,9,10] and up to 10% in Asian populations, especially the Chinese [5,6,8,11].

Table 3.4.1 Main characteristics of *SCA2* expansions in familial Parkinson's disease (PD) of different ethnic origins

Number of patients	Family origin	Inheritance	Parkinsonian triad	Response to levodopa	Ataxia	SCA2 expansion	Number of CAG repeats	Reference
136	Almost all Caucasians	AD	+	+	–	1.4%	33 and 35	3
270	Varied	96 familial	+	+	–	0%	–	4
242	Taiwan	Sporadic PD	+	+	–	0.4%	37	5
130	Taiwan	All familial (AD > AR)	+	+	In later stages	10%	35 to 38	6
280	Varied	114 familial (AD and AR)	+	+	–	2%	37	7
91	Singapore	All familial	+	+	–	1.1%	38	8
224	Italy	79 familial	+	+	–	1.2%	38	9
178	Europe (148)	AD	+	+	–	2%	37 and 39	10

AD, autosomal dominant; AR, autosomal recessive.

SCA2 expansions mimicking PD induce moderate symmetrical PD. Compared to our series of familial autosomal dominant PD patients, patients with *SCA2* expansions had fewer asymmetric symptoms ($P < 0.001$) on examination, a characteristic noted in previous studies [6], and less rigidity ($P < 0.01$). Despite similar disease durations, *SCA2* patients under treatment ("on") had lower UPDRS scores ($P < 0.01$), less frequent fluctuations ($P < 0.05$), and took less levodopa ($P < 0.05$). These observations are consistent with a recent study in Italian families where parkinsonism linked to *SCA2* mutation was described as benign [9].

SCA2 expansions mimicking PD are small and interrupted. In our three families, the expanded alleles had 37 to 39 repeats. This is in the lower range of *SCA2* expansions, and is consistent with previous reports in which most expansions in *SCA2* families with ADP had < 40 repeats [3,5,6,8,10–14]. The expansion size itself is not sufficient to explain the parkinsonian phenotype, as only 26% of ataxic patients with *SCA2* expansions in the same size range (35 to 39 repeats) had slight parkinsonian signs [10].

In *SCA2,* CAG repeat expansions inducing ataxic phenotypes are usually unstable upon transmission with a tendency to increase in size, resulting in phenotypic variability and anticipation of the age at onset [14]. In our series, the *SCA2* expansions differed in size, but all carried four CAA interruptions and were stably transmitted within each family [10]. These results suggest that the configuration of the *SCA2* CAG/CAA repeat expansions plays an important role in phenotypic variability.

SCA2 expansions mimicking PD have later onset than those with an ataxic phenotype. Onset of symptoms in *SCA2* patients with parkinsonism in our series occurred at age 50.1 ± 13.2 years vs. 35 ± 14 years for the ataxic phenotype. This difference in onset was not only the result of expansion size, because it persisted when we included only ataxic patients with the expansions in the same size range (44.4 ± 10.9 years). These results are consistent with those reported by Lu *et al.* [6], who found mean ages at onset of 47 and 27 years, respectively, for the parkinsonian and ataxic phenotypes, but no correlation with allele size.

Are there families with both ataxic and parkinsonian phenotypes? In the Chinese family described by Gwinn-Hardy *et al.* [11], both ataxic and parkinsonian phenotypes were present in the same family. Interestingly, the CAG repeat expansion was greater in the patient with an ataxic phenotype (43 CAG) than in the patients with parkinsonism (33, 35, or 36).

Parkinsonism is associated with nigral degeneration and striatal dysfunction. Brain MRI of *SCA2* patients with pure parkinsonism does not show cerebellar atrophy, at least in the early stages of the disease. Neuropathological examinations of ataxic *SCA2* cases have shown nigral degeneration with neuronal loss in the substantia nigra, striatum and pallidum [1,2]. Measurements of dopamine transporter and D2 receptor function using functional brain imaging have revealed striatal dysfunction [12,15], even in patients with an ataxic phenotype without parkinsonism [15].

Conclusion

Genetic factors play an important role in the pathogenesis of parkinsonism in young patients. Several genes have been implicated. *SCA2* expansions may manifest as typical parkinsonism. Although this is a rare cause of parkinsonism in Caucasians, a molecular analysis of *SCA2* should be included in genetic screening of families with dominant parkinsonism or patients with parkinsonism and family histories of neurodegenerative disorders.

Perrine Charles, Alexandra Dürr, Alexis Brice

References

1 Dürr A, Smadja D, Cancel G *et al.* Autosomal dominant cerebellar ataxia type I in Martinique (French West Indies): clinical and neuropathological analysis of 53 patients from three unrelated SCA2 families. *Brain* 1995; **118**: 1573–81.

2 Stevanin G, Dürr A, Brice A. Clinical and molecular advances in autosomal dominant cerebellar ataxias: from genotype to phenotype and physiopathology. *Eur J Hum Genet* 2000; **8**: 4–18.

3 Payami H, Nutt J, Gancher S *et al.* SCA2 may present as levodopa-responsive parkinsonism. *Mov Disord* 2003; **18**: 425–9.

4 Kock N, Muller B, Vieregge P *et al.* Role of SCA2 mutations in early- and late-onset dopa-responsive parkinsonism. *Ann Neurol* 2002; **52**: 257–8; author reply 258.

5 Shan DE, Liu RS, Sun CM, Lee SJ, Liao KK, Soong BW. Presence of spinocerebellar ataxia type 2 gene mutation in a patient with apparently sporadic Parkinson's disease: clinical implications. *Mov Disord* 2004; **19**: 1357–60.

6 Lu CS, Chang HC, Kuo PC *et al.* The parkinsonian phenotype of spinocerebellar ataxia type 2. *Arch Neurol* 2004; **61**: 35–8.

7 Simon-Sanchez J, Hanson M, Singleton A *et al.* Analysis of SCA-2 and SCA-3 repeats in Parkinsonism: evidence of SCA-2 expansion in a family with autosomal dominant Parkinson's disease. *Neurosci Lett* 2005; **382**: 1–8.

8 Lim SW, Zhao Y, Chua E *et al.* Genetic analysis of SCA2, 3 and 17 in idiopathic Parkinson's disease. *Neurosci Lett* 2006; **403**: 11–14.

9 Modoni A, Contarino MF, Bentivoglio AR *et al.* Prevalence of spinocerebellar ataxia type 2 mutation among Italian Parkinsonian patients. *Mov Disord* 2007; **22**(3): 324–7.

10 Charles P, Camuzat A, Benammar N *et al.* Are interrupted SCA2 CAG repeat expansions responsible for parkinsonism? *Neurology* 2007; Jun 13 [Epub ahead of print].

11 Gwinn-Hardy K, Chen JY, Liu HC *et al.* Spinocerebellar ataxia type 2 with parkinsonism in ethnic Chinese. *Neurology* 2000; **55**: 800–5.

12 Furtado S, Farrer M, Tsuboi Y, Klimek ML, de la Fuente-Fernandez R, Hussey J. SCA-2 presenting as parkinsonism in an Alberta family: clinical, genetic, and PET findings. *Neurology* 2002; **59**: 1625–7.

13 Furtado S, Payami H, Lockhart PJ, Hanson M, Nutt JG, Singleton AA. Profile of families with parkinsonism-predominant spinocerebellar ataxia type 2 (SCA2). *Mov Disord* 2004; **19**: 622–9.

14 Momeni P, Lu CS, Chou YH *et al.* Taiwanese cases of SCA2 are derived from a single founder. *Mov Disord* 2005; **20**: 1633–6.

15 Varrone A, Salvatore E, De Michele G *et al.* Reduced striatal [123 I]FP-CIT binding in SCA2 patients without parkinsonism. *Ann Neurol* 2004; **55**(3): 426–30.

Case study 5

Case presentation

A 39-year-old French woman was referred to our hospital for diagnosis and management of gait difficulties and memory decline.

Two years earlier, she had begun to have difficulty walking. She was troubled by forgetfulness and personality changes, often feeling depressed. On initial examination, her blinking rate was decreased and her facial expression, fixed. Her gait was shuffling, and arm swing was reduced bilaterally. Muscle strength was normal and she had brisk reflexes and bilateral ankle clonus. Plantar reflexes were flexor. Eye gaze was normal. There were no sensory or cerebellar signs and no tremor, myoclonus, or chorea. Cognitive functions were preserved, with normal performances in Luria's fist-edge-palm test.

The patient progressively developed symmetric rigidity and global bradykinesia, as well as mild dysarthria and swallowing difficulties. Limb hypertonia was mixed with both spastic and extrapyramidal features. Her gait became markedly impaired owing to axial rigidity and postural instability, with frequent backward falls. Levodopa therapy (250 mg, t.i.d.) had no impact on her rigid-akinetic syndrome. At age 45, she was unable to stand or walk without aid. She also showed progressive cognitive decline with severe executive dysfunction. Depression and behavioral changes became more prominent. During the 10-year follow-up, the patient never developed choreic movements and oculomotor examination remained normal. Brain magnetic resonance imaging (MRI), performed 9 years after onset, showed marked cortical atrophy and reduced size of caudate nuclei.

She had no personal medical history, but a positive family history. Her mother had progressive cognitive decline along with involuntary movements and died at the age of 38. Her brother had recently been diagnosed with Huntington disease (HD), confirmed by genetic analysis.

Differential diagnosis

The clinical diagnosis of a movement disorder combined with early cognitive features offers the opportunity to discuss a number of neurological disorders. Three main aspects can be highlighted in our patient: (1) a parkinsonian syndrome, (2) cognitive and mood dysfunction, and (3) family history of neurological disorders. The clue to the diagnosis of this case is the familial history of HD. It is important to note that clinical phenotypes among members of a single family can differ from one affected person to the other. Our patient's mother and brother had typical HD with chorea and cognitive decline, making the diagnosis possible in our patient even though her clinical presentation was very atypical.

Parkinsonism with a poor response to levodopa and cognitive/behavioral changes in a patient without a clear family history of neurological disorders might suggest a diagnosis of dementia with Lewy bodies (DLB). This condition is also characterized by visuospatial and dysexecutive symptoms with fluctuations in attention. The disease may start either with motor or cognitive symptoms. Importantly, the hiatus of < 1 year between the onset of both symptoms suggests this diagnosis. When parkinsonism is followed by dementia many years after disease onset, is it usually classified as PD with dementia (PDD). It is arguable that the distinction between DLB and PDD is theoretical and that these conditions are only different expressions of the same underlying disease process. PDD could have been a diagnostic consideration for our patient, were it not for the family history of neurological disorders.

Frontotemporal dementia (FTD) is a group of disorders in which cognitive symptoms may occur simultaneously with parkinsonism and motor neuron disease. The disease may be either sporadic or transmitted as an autosomal dominant trait with mutations in the tau (*MAPT*) or progranulin (*PGRN*) genes. Cognitive problems may manifest as language disorder (semantic dementia or primary progressive aphasia) or a frontal syndrome with personality changes, memory decline, and disinhibition. A hyperkinetic syndrome, however, as presented by the patient's mother, makes this diagnostic very unlikely.

Parkinsonism with poor response to levodopa, oculomotor abnormalities, and frequent backward falls early on in the disease course suggest a diagnosis of progressive supranuclear palsy (PSP). Although our patient developed postural instability later in the disease course, eye movement abnormalities were never detected.

In all the conditions described above, levodopa has a minimal impact on parkinsonian symptoms. Drug-induced parkinsonism with depression can be seen in some countries where medications such as cinnarizine and flunarizine are sold over the counter to palliate vestibular symptoms.

Five to ten per cent of Parkinson's disease cases are transmitted as an autosomal dominant or recessive trait. In the small proportion of families in which a specific mutation in a single gene can be found, phenotypes range from mild parkinsonism with slow disease progression and prolonged response to levodopa to phenotypes indistinguishable from sporadic PD.

In all the cases above, the diagnosis is clinical and can only occasionally be aided by supplementary methods. Neuropsychological examination with tests that indicate cortical (predominant memory loss) and specific subcortical (predominant attention deficits) involvements are usually recommended. In FTD, imaging may disclose frontal and anterior or posterior temporal atrophy. Functional imaging studies (fMRI, PET, and SPECT) are useful as research tools, but still need numerous methodological improvements before being considered for clinical practice. Molecular analyses are possible for some families with FTD, for which we now know of disease-causing mutations in at least two genes. In PD, 11 different loci have been ascribed for autosomal dominant and recessive modes of transmission. In the case of positive screening, this allows adequate genetic counseling to be given to all family members.

The combination of cognitive decline, parkinsonism, *and* a family history of involuntary movements leaves little doubt as to the diagnosis of Huntington disease.

Final diagnosis: PD-mimicking Huntington disease confirmed by the presence of one allele with an abnormally expanded CAG trinucleotide stretch with 46 repeats in the *HD1* gene on chromosome 4.

Discussion

This diagnosis would not have been so evident had the patient's family history not been obtained. This is mandatory in current Movement Disorder guidelines. The disease usually starts with behavioral and personality changes, followed by chorea. In fact, executive and memory changes may be detected in otherwise asymptomatic mutation carriers [1]. Moreover, the personality changes are even more stereotyped and recognizable than the cognitive features. In individuals displaying the full HD clinical picture, cognitive changes correlate with atrophy of the striatum, thalamus and frontal lobes. Decreased striatal metabolism also parallels cognitive impairment [2]. Postmortem evaluation of patients with overt dementia shows accumulation of neocortical ubiquitin-reactive neurites [3].

Parkinsonism at onset in HD is typically seen in young patients with large trinucleotide expansions (>60 repeats). This was traditionally referred to as the Westphal variant of HD. A recent retrospective study showed that parkinsonism is not the main feature of juvenile HD, but that cognitive difficulties occur early in the disease course [4]. Bradykinesia and rigidity are also detected in individuals with "classic" HD, in whom chorea predominates the clinical picture, and may correlate with the degree of neostriatal degeneration better than chorea [5]. It is not clear to what extent decreased dopamine plays a role in HD-related parkinsonism [6,7].

In summary, this case illustrates the notion that parkinsonism can be the presenting feature of HD later in life and not only during adolescence and early adulthood. As is true with other forms of parkinsonism-plus, the patient being evaluated for parkinsonism may present with "red flags" of cognitive decline and unsatisfactory response to levodopa. Cognitive and/or personality changes may be noticeably more prominent than in the typical presentation of idiopathic PD. Finally, we suggest adopting a high level of suspicion for HD in individuals with early-onset atypical parkinsonism, particularly if there is a family history of movement disorders and even in its absence, as the lack of appropriate genealogical information can limit the evaluation of inherited disorders.

André R. Troiano, Leorah Freeman, Alexandra Dürr

References

1 Hahn-Barma V, Deweer B, Durr A *et al.* Are cognitive changes the first symptoms of Huntington's disease? A study of gene carriers. *J Neurol Neurosurg Psychiatry* 1998; **64**: 172–7.

2 Berent S, Giordani B, Lehtinen S *et al.* Positron emission tomographic scan investigations of Huntington's disease: cerebral metabolic correlates of cognitive function. *Ann Neurol* 1988; **23**: 541–6.

3 Cammarata S, Caponnetto C, Tabaton M. Ubiquitin-reactive neurites in cerebral cortex of subjects with Huntington's chorea: a pathological correlate of dementia? *Neurosci Lett* 1993; **156**: 96–8.

4 Ribai P, Nguyen K, Hahn-Barma V *et al.* Psychiatric and cognitive difficulties as indicators of juvenile Huntington disease onset in 29 patients. *Arch Neurol* 2007; **64**: 813–19.

5 Sanchez-Pernaute R, Kunig G, del Barrio Alba A *et al.* Bradykinesia in early Huntington's disease. *Neurology* 2000; **54**: 119–25.

6 Garcia Ruiz PJ, Mena MA, Sanchez Bernardos V *et al.* Cerebrospinal fluid homovanillic acid is reduced in untreated Huntington's disease. *Clin Neuropharmacol* 1995; **18**: 58–63.

7 Kurlan R, Goldblatt D, Zaczek R *et al.* Cerebrospinal fluid homovanillic acid and parkinsonism in Huntington's disease. *Ann Neurol* 1988; **24**: 282–4.

Case study 6

Case presentation

A 52-year-old right-handed male with no significant past medical history developed progressive pain in his right shoulder.

He had been in his usual state of good health until 6 months before presentation, when he developed increasing pain in his right shoulder. He described soreness and stiffness that worsened with movement. He also reported that his range of motion was slightly restricted. He continued to work without limitation as a sales manager, but felt tired. In the last few months, he had begun taking a nap on the weekends. His wife reported that his sleep had deteriorated over the last few years, citing occasional nightmares and thrashing. He also described mild symptoms of depression, and his family added that he had become "irritable" and mildly withdrawn, being quieter than usual. The patient reported that his handwriting had become smaller but was legible. He also noted that sometimes his thumb would "twitch."

The patient was seen by his family physician, who made a clinical diagnosis of rotator cuff injury. The patient took ibuprofen 600 mg t.i.d. for 3 weeks with some improvement in his shoulder pain. Laboratory studies included normal complete blood count, electrolyte panel, liver function, thyroid-stimulating hormone, and sedimentation rate. Radiographs of the shoulder were normal.

On general examination the patient appeared well. His vital signs and general condition were normal. He demonstrated a mildly depressed mood and blunted affect. He scored 29/30 on the Mini Mental State Examination (losing one point for recall). His language function was normal. His speech was soft, with a mild hypokinetic dysarthria. His cranial nerve examination was normal, including full extraocular, saccadic, and smooth pursuit eye movements. His motor examination demonstrated normal bulk and strength throughout. He had mild cogwheel rigidity in the right arm, with activation of the left arm; otherwise his tone was normal. When distracted, an intermittent, low frequency resting tremor was noted in the right thumb. This was also evident while walking. His reflexes were normal and symmetrical. No pathological reflexes were noted. His sensory exam was normal to touch, pinprick, temperature, joint position sense, and vibration. Cortical reflexes were intact, with normal graphesthesias and stereographia. His coordination was normal and he did not demonstrate apraxia. His gait was notable for slightly decreased right arm swing. Pull test was negative. A writing sample demonstrated subtle micrographia. His UPSIT (University of Pennsylvania Smell Identification Test) score was 23/40.

Differential diagnosis

The differential diagnosis for this patient largely revolves around parkinsonism. He has monomelic involvement of the right arm characterized by resting tremor, cogwheel rigidity, bradykinesia (decreased arm swing), and subsequent shoulder pain. Other subtle features of his history and examination support this, including micrographia and hypophonia. The asymmetrical findings, in conjunction with microsmia, support a likely diagnosis of Parkinson's disease (PD). He has other associated features including fatigue, depression, and rapid eye movement (REM) sleep behavior disorder (RBD).

Other causes of parkinsonism should be considered. There is no history to suggest a secondary cause of parkinsonism. The asymmetrical nature of this patient's symptoms would make drug or toxin-induced causes, normal pressure hydrocephalus, or metabolic diseases such as Wilson's disease or neurodegeneration with brain iron accumulation (NBIA-1), unlikely causes of his parkinsonism. There is no history to suggest an infectious process. A structural, left-sided basal ganglia mass lesion could cause focal parkinsonism. It would be unusual, however, to find parkinsonism in isolation, without any other neurological deficits or exam abnormalities. Similarly, vascular parkinsonism is possible, but unlikely in this young, otherwise healthy patient.

Atypical parkinsonian syndromes can also be considered, but are unlikely given the history and clinical findings. These degenerative disorders often have accompanying features that this patient lacks. Progressive supranuclear palsy (PSP) can present with parkinsonism, but vertical gaze palsy and postural instability are also usually present. Corticobasal degeneration (CBD) can present with asymmetrical parkinsonism, but is characterized by limb apraxia, and ultimately alien limb syndrome. Furthermore, CBD and PSP typically do not have tremor. If prominent autonomic or cerebellar symptoms were present, multiple system atrophy (MSA) could be considered. Patients suffering from dementia with Lewy bodies (DLB) or Alzheimer's disease (AD) can present parkinsonism and depression, but these disorders are characterized by prominent cognitive dysfunction which usually overshadows motor symptoms. DLB can also involve fluctuating mental status, visual hallucinations and significant sleep disturbance (RBD). Frontotemporal dementia parkinsonism is unlikely given the absence of dementia.

Shoulder pain is often of musculoskeletal origin. Joint disease is a common cause of asymmetrical pain and/or loss of movement, as are osteoarthritis, tendonitis, and bursitis. A cervical radiculopathy can also result in shoulder pain. These diagnoses, however, would only explain our patient's pain and not his other symptoms. Although chronic pain can cause depression, rigidity and tremor would not be expected. Therefore, these pathologies alone would not provoke his symptoms.

Parkinson's disease is largely a clinical diagnosis. Adjunctive testing, however, can further support this conclusion in lieu of a definitive pathological diagnosis. Magnetic resonance imaging (MRI) of the brain would rule out structural or vascular causes, which are particularly important if findings are unilateral or abrupt in onset. An MRI is not generally necessary if symptoms are typical. In idiopathic PD, one would expect a normal MRI of the brain. Olfactory deficits can precede motor deficits in PD. Therefore, smell testing may be a sensitive screening tool for early PD [1]. However, because this is non-specific, other testing can be helpful. If Wilson's disease is suspected, serum and urine copper levels, plasma ceruloplasmin levels and a slit-lamp exam (to rule out Keyser–Fleischer rings) are indicated.

Although not performed routinely, cardiac sympathetic imaging studies using ^{123}I-MIBG (meta-iodobenzylguanidine) scintigraphy may also prove useful in differentiating idiopathic PD from PSP and MSA [2]. In preliminary studies, patients with PD demonstrated cardiac sympathetic denervation while patients with PSP and MSA did not. PD patients also have visual abnormalities including deficits in contrast sensitivity and color discrimination [3]. Prolonged visual evoked potential latencies can be seen as well [4]. Whether these novel tests of other non-motor systems become useful in medical practice, particularly in early or even premotor disease, will be determined by further research.

Neuroimaging may also prove useful in the diagnosis of early PD. Fluoro-dopa positron emission tomography (PET) and 2β-carbomethoxy-3β-(4-iodophenyl)tropane (β-CIT) single photon emission computed tomography (SPECT) are useful if the diagnosis of PD is in doubt. Research is under way to determine the utility of PET and SPECT both as a preclinical diagnostic tool and as a means of determining progression of nigrostriatal dysfunction in PD [5,6].

Final diagnosis: early Parkinson's disease.

Discussion

The cardinal signs and symptoms of Parkinson's disease are well recognized in the medical community: resting tremor, bradykinesia, and rigidity. Less recognized, however, are the more subtle or early features of PD. Early clinical features of motor involvement can be slight and initially attributed to normal aging. It is common for patients to reflect on early symptoms that went unrecognized. Bradykinesia can manifest as a loss of spontaneous movement, such as reduced arm swing, loss of facial expressivity, or subtle changes in speech volume or clarity. Loss of manual dexterity is also an early sign. Patients may report difficulty doing up buttons, or deterioration in their handwriting. Pain, in general, can be an early and common symptom of PD. This may be a function of musculoskeletal discomfort from rigidity, dystonia, or lack of movement, or present as a primary pain syndrome. This symptom often leads to a musculoskeletal diagnosis, as in this case.

Presymptomatic and non-motor features of Parkinson's disease are gaining support as preclinical markers or risk factors for PD [7]. Loss of smell, behavioral abnormalities, fatigue, sleep disorders, and autonomic dysfunction are all now recognized as presymptomatic or early features of PD. Depression, anxiety, and personality changes can precede motor symptoms and are common in PD [8,9]. It is not unusual for patients to experience RBD years prior to onset of motor PD symptoms [10]. Similarly, many PD patients report autonomic dysfunction, often constipation [11], which also can predate motor symptoms by years. Although non-specific, these non-motor symptoms can often be used to add confidence to the clinical diagnosis of PD. In the future these symptoms may enable clinicians to identify at-risk populations in which to ultimately apply neuroprotective strategies [12].

Jayne R. Wilkinson, Matthew B. Stern

References

1 Ponsen MM, Stoffers D, Booij J, van Eck-Smit BL, Wolters ECh, Berendese HW. Idiopathic hyposmia as a preclinical sign of Parkinson's disease. *Ann Neurol* 2004; **56**(2): 173–81.

2 Yoshita M. Differentiation of idiopathic Parkinson's disease from striatonigral degeneration and progressive supranuclear palsy using iodine-123 and metaiodobenzylguanidine myocardial scintigraphy. *J Neurol Sci* 1998; **155**: 60–6.

3 Pieri V, Diederich NJ, Raman R, Goetz CG. Decreased color discrimination and contrast sensitivity in Parkinson's disease. *J Neurol Sci* 2000; **172**(1): 7–11.

4 Bodis-Wollner I, Yahr MD. Measurement of visual evoked potentials in Parkinson's disease, *Brain* 1978; **101**: 661–71.

5 Brucke T, Asenbaum S, Pirker W *et al.* Measurement of the dopaminergic degeneration in Parkinson's disease with [^{123}I]β-CIT and SPECT. *J Neural Transm Suppl* 1997; **50**: 9–224.

6 Scherfler C, Schwarz J, Antonini A *et al.* Role of DAT-SPECT in the diagnostic work up of Parkinsonism. *Mov Disord* 2007; **22**(9): 1229–38.

7 Tolosa E, Compta Y, Gaig C. The premotor phase of Parkinson's disease. *Parkinsonism Relat Disord* 2007; **13**(Suppl 1): S2–7.

8 Ishihara L, Brayne C. A systematic review of depression and mental illness preceding Parkinson's disease. *Acta Neurol Scand* 2006; **113**: 211–20.

9 Weintraub D, Stern MB. Psychiatric complications in Parkinson's disease. *Am J Geriatr Psychiatry* 2005; **13**: 844–51.

10 Postuma RB, Lang AE, Massicotte-Marquez J, Montplaisir. Potential early markers of Parkinson's disease in idiopathic REM sleep behavior disorder. *Neurology* 2006; **66**(6): 845–51.

11 Edwards LL, Pfeiffer RF, Quigley EMM, Hofman R, Baluff M. Gastrointestinal symptoms in Parkinson's disease. *Mov Disord* 1991; **6**: 151–6.

12 Abbott RD, Ross GW, White LR *et al.* Environmental, life-style, and physical precursors of clinical Parkinson's disease: recent findings from the Honolulu-Asia Aging Study. *J Neurol* 2003; **250**: III30–9.

Case study 7

Case presentation

A 62-year-old woman presented at our movement disorders clinic following 3 years of progressive gait problems. Since the beginning, she had noticed some general slowing of her movements and an intermittent tremor of both arms, which mainly occurred during movement or while holding an object. She described her arm and hand movements as slow and of small amplitude, rendering the activities of daily living difficult. Some falls had occurred and she complained of an increasingly bent-forward posture. Since the previous year, urinary stress incontinence had appeared on different occasions. Recently, urinary urge incontinence had also been noticed. She had always slept well and nightmares were rare. Her husband, who attended with her, did not report snoring, signs of sleep apnea, or nocturnal stridor, but had observed some motor agitation and his wife talking in her sleep. According to the patient and her husband, there were no relevant mood or memory disturbances. The family history was negative for neurodegenerative diseases and the patient had no relevant pre-existing medical condition.

Following disease onset, the patient had been treated with Requip® (ropinirole) up to 16 mg per day, with only a minor improvement in her symptoms. Requip® had been replaced with 150 mg Stalevo® five times per day (levodopa 150 mg/carbidopa 37.5 mg/entacapone 200 mg) and 100 mg Sinemet® five times per day (levodopa 100 mg/carbidopa 10 mg) during the second year of her disease.

The neurological examination showed saccadic horizontal and vertical pursuit eye movements without any other signs of oculomotor dysfunction. Mild to moderate dysarthria and hypomimia were observed. Finger-tapping and foot-tapping revealed moderate bradykinesia, predominantly on the left. Rigidity was moderate in the left arm and only mild in the right arm and neck. The patient had bilateral postural tremor that was only present while counting. Her posture was slightly bent forward. Gait was wide-based, slow and unstable, with reduced step length and difficulties while turning. Automatic movements of the left arm were reduced while walking. Stance became more unstable when joining both feet and she would have fallen during the tandem Romberg maneuver had she not been helped. Postural responses were moderately impaired. Limb dysmetria was absent. No sensorimotor deficit could be detected. Tendon reflexes were very brisk but symmetrical and plantar responses were flexor. She had a Mini Mental State Examination score of 27/30 and frontal lobe testing only revealed minor disturbances. Testing for orthostatic hypotension was normal.

In her diagnostic work-up, the patient underwent cerebral magnetic resonance imaging (MRI) which revealed a hyperintense rim of the right putamen on T2-weighted imaging and a putaminal hypointensity on T2*-weighted gradient echo images (Fig. 3.7.1). Testing of bladder function revealed a postmicturition residual volume of 220 mL, detrusor hyperreflexia during the filling phase causing urinary leakage, and detrusor-external sphincter dyssynergia during the voiding phase.

Differential diagnosis

Parkinson's disease (PD) is characterized by an asymmetrical bradykinetic-rigid syndrome. Although postural instability with falls is common after several years of PD, the signs of cerebellar impairment in our patient exclude the clinical diagnosis of PD. Autonomic dysfunction exists in PD, but it is usually less severe and the motor symptoms respond to dopaminergic treatment, in contrast to the present case.

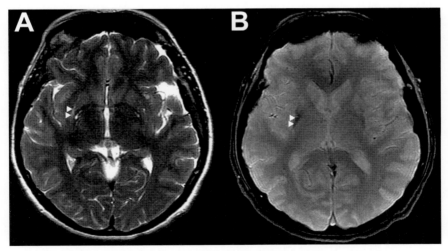

Figure 3.7.1 MRI of the patient's brain. (A) T2-weighted imaging; white arrowheads, hyperintensive rim of the right putamen. (B) T2*-weighted gradient echo images; white arrowheads, putaminal hypointensity.

Parkinsonism can also be found in frontotemporal dementia, Lewy body dementia, and Alzheimer's disease. The cognitive decline in these patients, however, is prominent whereas our patient's cognitive functions remained intact.

Patients presenting progressive supranuclear palsy (PSP) show a vertical supranuclear palsy or at least slowing of vertical saccades, as well as prominent postural instability with frequent falls. Supportive features of PSP are early cognitive impairment such as apathy, impairment in abstract thought, decreased verbal fluency, utilization or imitation behavior, or frontal release signs. Findings on MRI and functional imaging mainly show a reduced midbrain diameter and frontotemporal atrophy. The response to dopaminergic treatment is usually poor and transient, as in our patient. The diagnosis of PSP is unlikely, however, since the clinical exam did not find a supranuclear palsy, and furthermore postural instability was not a major feature despite some falls in the past.

Patients suffering from corticobasal degeneration (CBD) have asymmetrical parkinsonism. Asymmetrical limb dystonia is common, often evolving to a painful "dystonic clenched fist." Higher cortical dysfunction such as aphasia, ideomotor or constructive apraxia, sensory abnormalities, an alien-limb phenomenon, and frontal lobe release signs belong to the clinical features of CBD. Cortical atrophy is more severe in CBD compared to other movement disorders. The response to dopaminergic treatment is usually poor and transient. Our patient had asymmetrical parkinsonism with poor levodopa-response, but did not show signs of higher cortical dysfunction, ruling out the clinical diagnosis of CBD.

Spinocerebellar ataxia 3 can resemble PD, but patients usually have a family history of dominant inheritance and show other symptoms such as a cerebellar syndrome, pyramidal signs, supranuclear vertical gaze palsy, and sometimes lower motor neuron disease with amyotrophy and fasciculations.

Multiple system atrophy (MSA) is associated with autonomic failure, parkinsonism, cerebellar dysfunction, and pyramidal signs. Other clinical signs such as orofacial dystonia, nocturnal stridor, sleep apnea, and rapid eye movement (REM) sleep behavior disorder (RBD) may also be found. The response to dopaminergic treatment is usually poor and transient. In Western countries, a predominantly parkinsonian phenotype (MSA-P) is present in two-thirds of patients, while one-third shows a predominant cerebellar phenotype (MSA-C).

Final diagnosis: multiple system atrophy.

Discussion

Our patient's poorly levodopa-responsive asymmetrical parkinsonian syndrome with signs of cerebellar impairment and bladder dysfunction is in line with the diagnostic criteria of "probable" MSA [1]. These define "probable" MSA as reaching the criterion for autonomic failure (orthostatic fall in blood pressure by at least 30 mmHg systolic or 15 mmHg diastolic) and/or urinary incontinence (persistent, involuntary partial or total bladder emptying, accompanied by erectile dysfunction) plus poorly levodopa-responsive parkinsonism (bradykinesia plus rigidity, postural instability, or tremor) or cerebellar dysfunction (gait ataxia plus ataxic dysarthria, limb ataxia, or sustained gaze-evoked nystagmus). The diagnosis further distinguishes between "possible" MSA with a lower degree of clinical evidence and "definite" MSA, the latter being the postmortem confirmation of typical α-synuclein-containing intracytoplasmic glial inclusions.

The clinical diagnosis of MSA is further supported by the findings of cerebral MRI showing a hyperintense rim of the right putamen on T2-weighted images and a putaminal hypointensity on T2*-weighted gradient echo images. These findings are frequent in patients with MSA-P and are indicative of reactive microgliosis, astrogliosis, and iron deposition [2,3]. In patients with MSA-C, olivopontocerebellar atrophy, the so-called hot-cross bun sign (cross-shaped signal hyperintensity on T2-weighted sequences within the pons), and atrophy of the middle cerebral peduncle may be found on MRI [3]. Diffusion-weighted imaging with calculation of the apparent diffusion coefficient can be useful in distinguishing MSA from other movement disorders such as PD [4].

The patient had a postmicturition residual volume of >200 mL, detrusor hyperreflexia during the filling phase, and detrusor-external sphinter dyssynergia during the voiding phase. Bladder dysfunction can be seen in PD, but is usually less frequent, less severe, and occurs at later stages of the disease. Detrusor hyperreflexia during the filling phase is more common in PD than in MSA [5]. A residual volume of >100 mL, however, has a positive predictive value of 91.6% for MSA [6], and detrusor-external sphincter dyssynergia is observed in 50% of MSA patients, while absent in PD [5]. The performance of an external urethral or anal sphincter electromyography can be useful in the differential diagnosis, since it shows denervation in MSA, but not in PD [7,8].

No signs of orthostatic hypotension were observed. Cardiovascular autonomic function can be assessed by the Ewing test battery. This comprises the measurement of the variability of arterial blood pressure and heart rate after standing up and during sustained isometric handgrip, as well as the assessment of heart-rate variability during deep breathing and the Valsalva maneuver.

Tests that are useful to distinguish autonomic failure in MSA from PD are cardiac ^{123}I-metaiodobenzylguanidine (MIBG) SPECT [9] and the arginine-growth hormone test [10]. MIBG SPECT shows impaired MIBG uptake in PD but not in MSA, in line with postganglionic autonomic failure in PD and the degeneration of preganglionic sympathetic fibers in MSA.

It is probable that, in line with her husband's description, the patient also presents RBD which is present in almost all patients suffering from MSA [11]. By contrast, no signs of sleep apnea or nocturnal stridor were reported. Since

Table 3.7.1 "Red flag" signs (modified according to Wenning *et al.* [11])

"Red flag" signs
Rapid progression with positive "wheelchair" sign within 5 years of disease onset
Orofacial dystonia or dyskinesia
Disproportionate antecollis
Pisa syndrome (lateral flexion of the trunk)
Camptocormia
Contractures of hands or feet
Jerky tremor
Severe dysarthria and/or dysphagia
Nocturnal or diurnal inspiratory stridor, inspiratory sighs, sleep apnea, excessive snoring
REM sleep behavior disorder
Raynaud's phenomenon, cold hands or feet
Emotional incontinence (crying or laughing)

these are frequent in MSA and probably related to a poorer outcome [12], they should be looked for systematically.

In conclusion, the clinical diagnosis of MSA is based on the association of autonomic failure plus poorly levodopa-responsive parkinsonism and/or cerebellar dysfunction. Additional paraclinical tests such as MRI, autonomic function tests, and sphincter electromyography may be helpful to endorse the diagnosis of MSA. The differential diagnosis between PD and MSA-P can be very difficult in early stages of the disease, mainly when MSA-P patients respond to dopaminergic treatment, as seen in 10–30% [11]. In these patients, the presence of other clinical features, the so-called "red flags" (Table 3.7.1), should orient the diagnosis towards MSA-P.

Wassilios Meissner, François Tison

References

1 Gilman S, Low PA, Quinn N *et al.* Consensus statement on the diagnosis of multiple system atrophy. *J Neurol Sci* 1999; **163**(1): 94–8.
2 Kraft E, Trenkwalder C, Auer DP. T2*-weighted MRI differentiates multiple system atrophy from Parkinson's disease. *Neurology* 2002; **59**(8): 1265–7.
3 Schrag A, Good CD, Miszkiel K *et al.* Differentiation of atypical parkinsonian syndromes with routine MRI. *Neurology* 2000; **54**(3): 697–702.
4 Nicoletti G, Lodi R, Condino F *et al.* Apparent diffusion coefficient measurements of the middle cerebellar peduncle differentiate the Parkinson variant of MSA from Parkinson's disease and progressive supranuclear palsy. *Brain* 2006; **129**(Pt 10): 2679–87.
5 Sakakibara R, Hattori T, Uchiyama T, Yamanishi T. Videourodynamic and sphincter motor unit potential analyses in Parkinson's disease and multiple system atrophy. *J Neurol Neurosurg Psychiatry* 2001; **71**(5): 600–6.
6 Hahn K, Ebersbach G. Sonographic assessment of urinary retention in multiple system atrophy and idiopathic Parkinson's disease. *Mov Disord* 2005; **20**(11): 1499–1502.
7 Palace J, Chandiramani VA, Fowler CJ. Value of sphincter electromyography in the diagnosis of multiple system atrophy. *Muscle Nerve* 1997; **20**(11): 1396–1403.

8 Beck RO, Betts CD, Fowler CJ. Genitourinary dysfunction in multiple system atrophy: clinical features and treatment in 62 cases. *J Urol* 1994; **151**(5): 1336–41.

9 Braune S, Reinhardt M, Schnitzer R, Riedel A, Lucking CH. Cardiac uptake of [123I] MIBG separates Parkinson's disease from multiple system atrophy. *Neurology* 1999; **53**(5): 1020–5.

10 Pellecchia MT, Longo K, Pivonello R *et al*. Multiple system atrophy is distinguished from idiopathic Parkinson's disease by the arginine growth hormone stimulation test. *Ann Neurol* 2006; **60**(5): 611–15.

11 Wenning GK, Colosimo C, Geser F, Poewe W. Multiple system atrophy. *Lancet Neurol* 2004; **3**(2): 93–103.

12 Silber MH, Levine S. Stridor and death in multiple system atrophy. *Mov Disord* 2000; **15**(4): 699–704.

Case study 8

Case presentation

A 65-year-old right-handed white female with a college education complained of balance and visual disturbances. She presented with a 3-year history of progressive postural instability and falls. Initially, she would fall back into the chair when attempting to get up. Later she began to fall when reaching for something, and now she was falling once or twice a day when walking unaided.

For the past 2 years looking up had progressively become difficult, and lately, also looking down and reading. For approximately 2 years, she had suffered from progressive dysphagia, from dysarthria for the past 6 months, and from slowness and emotional lability. She denied urinary or orthostatic hypotension symptoms. She was taking aspirin once per day and had never taken dopaminergic therapy. She had undergone partial thyroidectomy. Family history was non-contributory.

General examination of the patient was normal, with no signs of orthostatic hypotension. The patient was alert, oriented to time, person, and space. Her Mini Mental Status Examination score was 25/30 (owing to attention errors). Mattis Dementia Rating Scale was 120/144 (mild dementia); she had conceptualization, attention, and construction errors. Frontal lobe function testing showed a lack of conceptualization, difficulty with sequencing, and decreased verbal fluency. There were no ideomotor apraxia, cortical sensory deficits, or language disturbances.

Cranial nerves were normal except for the presence of limited upward more than downward voluntary gaze, absence of vertical saccades, and optokinetic nystagmus. Pursuit and vestibular reflex in the vertical direction were preserved. Horizontal saccades were slow but there was no limitation in horizontal voluntary or pursuit gaze. Horizontal optokinetic nystagmus was normal. There was no convergence. Her blink rate was decreased and she had hypomimia and slight staring face.

Motor examination showed full strength. Tone was increased axially more than distally. Bradykinesia was more axial than in the limb muscles. No tremor, dystonia, or myoclonus were observed. She had normal deep tendon reflexes, and downgoing plantar reflexes. Sensory examination was normal.

The patient was unable to get up from her chair without holding onto the arms. When sitting down, she tended to let herself fall into the chair. Her gait was wide-based and unstable, requiring a walker. Furthermore, she would fall with the pull test unless assisted by the examiner. Finally, coordination was normal.

Differential diagnosis

Our patient presented at 62 years of age with postural instability and falls, followed by vertical supranuclear gaze palsy, parkinsonism affecting axial more than limb muscles, dysarthia, dysphagia, and frontal lobe-type features. She presented with all the typical features of progressive supranuclear palsy (PSP) and meets the clinically definite criteria for this disorder [1]. The main inclusion criteria for the diagnosis of clinically definite PSP is the presence after age 40 of progressive vertical supranuclear gaze palsy, severe postural instability, and falls within the first year of symptom onset. Mandatory exclusion criteria include lack of severe lateralized motor signs or ideomotor apraxia, autonomic features, oculomasticatory myorrhythmia, and structural lesions revealed by magnetic resonance imaging (MRI).

Our patient's first symptom, severe postural instability, manifested as non-explained and unexpected falls or tendency to fall. This is the most frequent symptom in PSP. Unexplained postural instability and falls occurring within the first year of symptom onset makes PSP the most likely diagnosis [2]. When falls occur after the first year, multiple system atrophy (MSA) is equally possible; however, instability and falls in MSA are usually present once patients already exhibit autonomic disturbances. Instability or falls rarely develop early in patients with corticobasal syndrome (CBS) that may associate with corticobasal degeneration. When they occur, they are usually due to unilateral limb involvement, a feature not observed in our patient. In Parkinson's disease (PD), falls are not an early feature; however, falls may occur early in dementia with Lewy bodies (DLB), and usually are associated with early cognitive disturbances and hallucinations that are not drug-related.

In our patient, the presence of vertical supranuclear gaze palsy allows the diagnosis of PSP to be made. Vertical supranuclear gaze palsy is rarely present at symptom onset; it usually takes 3–4 years to develop. Slowing of saccades (distinctly slowed eye movements when attempting to move the eyes rapidly between two stimuli) usually precedes the development of the supranuclear gaze palsy, and allows for an earlier diagnosis of the disease. Our patient also exhibited slowing of horizontal saccades, usually preceding the development of the horizontal supranuclear gaze palsy.

Although key in diagnosing PSP, vertical supranuclear palsy may occasionally be present in patients with DLB, arteriosclerotic pseudoparkinsonism, CBS, Creutzfeldt–Jakob disease, or Whipple's disease. Symptom progression, however, is usually helpful to differentiate between these disorders. In PSP, as in our patient, vertical supranuclear gaze palsy precedes the development of the horizontal gaze palsy. In CBS, ocular motor apraxia usually precedes the development of supranuclear gaze palsy which usually affects both horizontal and vertical gaze. The saccades in CBS may have an increased latency but normal speed, and are similarly affected in the vertical and horizontal plane, whereas in MSA the saccades have normal speed and latency. In our patient, the upward gaze palsy was the first indication of an ocular motor abnormality. This may need to be differentiated from the limitation of upward gaze observed in elderly patients, which is associated with normal saccades. The diagnosis in our patient did not require this distinction as she had no vertical saccades or optokinetic nystagmus on examination and had some downward gaze limitation. She also exhibited a profoundly sparse blink rate, typical of PSP. Although blink rate is often diminished in PD and MSA, this is usually to a lesser degree than in PSP.

Our patient also presented with symmetric parkinsonism involving axial muscles more than limb muscles, a characteristic typically observed in patients with PSP. Patients with PD, DLB, or CBS usually have more limb than axial involvement, and the limb involvement is usually asymmetric. She also presented with speech and swallowing difficulties within the first 3 years of symptom onset. Prominent early or severe dysarthria may also be present in CBS and MSA, but is rare in PD.

She also exhibited frontal lobe symptomatology manifested by attentional disturbances, difficulty with conceptualization and sequencing, and decreased verbal fluency, features usually present at early stages in PSP. Executive dysfunction of PSP patients also manifests as difficulty with planning and problem solving. Frontal behavioral disturbances (primarily apathy, but also disinhibition) are also frequent. Frontal lobe features in PD and MSA are usually mild, and revealed only through detailed neuropsychological testing, in contrast to what is observed in PSP. Because patients with PSP usually exhibit early frontal lobe cognitive and/or behavioral disturbances, they occasionally are confused with patients with frontal dementia or Alzheimer's disease [3]. However in PSP, features of "cortical" dementia are rare or only mild, unless the patient also suffers from Alzheimer's disease. Our patient did not exhibit either the lateralized cognitive features (unilateral ideomotor apraxia, cortical sensory signs, or aphasia) observed in patients with CBS. Finally, she did not exhibit autonomic signs (e.g. incontinence or presyncope) or cerebellar disturbances suggestive of MSA.

The diagnosis of PSP in our patient is obvious for clinicians familiar with this condition. Infrequently, however, PSP may be associated with unusual traits, which make the diagnosis of this disorder more challenging. There are reports of neuropathologically confirmed cases of PSP with parkinsonism that respond to dopaminergic medication and lack ophthalmoplegia (PSP-parkinsonism); with dementia or akinesia as the only presenting symptom; with unilateral dystonia and apraxia; or with motor aphasia and speech apraxia [4].

Survival in patients such as ours who present with all the typical features of PSP within the first 2 years of symptom onset is around 5 years. Early falls, supranuclear gaze palsy, and dysphagia are predictors of a shorter survival in several studies.

Final diagnosis: progressive supranuclear palsy.

Discussion

Presently, there are no biological markers for the diagnosis of PSP; this is usually a clinical diagnosis eventually confirmed by pathology. Neuropsychological evaluation is particularly helpful to support the diagnosis since, as in our patient, almost all PSP patients examined demonstrate an early and prominent difficulty in executive dysfunction. Similarly, apathy but not depression is usually present early in patients with PSP and can be easily identified by using the Neuropsychiatric Inventory.

Brain MRI may show definite atrophy of the midbrain and of the region around the third ventricle in PSP patients. Thinning of the quadrigeminal plate, particularly in its superior part, better seen in sagittal MRI sections, supports a diagnosis of PSP. Minimal signal abnormalities in the periaqueductal region may also be seen in proton density MRI. Brain MRI can also aid in ruling out other diagnoses (e.g. multi-infarct states, hydrocephalus, or tumors, as well as MSA when atrophy of the pons, middle cerebellar peduncles, and cerebellum, or altered signal intensity in the putamen are observed).

Transcranial sonography (TCS) may be able to differentiate PSP from other parkinsonian disorders [5]. TCS in PSP shows characteristic changes such as abnormal hyperechogenicity of the lenticular nucleus and normal echogenicity of the substantia nigra. In contrast, patients with PD have hyperechogenicity of the substantia nigra and normal echogenicity of the lenticular nuclei. Lenticular nuclei hyperechogenicity is also observed in MSA, but dilation of the third ventricule (> 10 mm) so far has been only described in PSP. TCS can differentiate PSP from CBD as the latter has markedly increased echogenicity of the substantia nigra.

Currently, there are no effective therapies that slow disease progression but symptoms can be ameliorated, and close follow-up can help prevent complications. Our patient should try dopaminergic medication, although the majority of PSP patients usually have an absent, poor, or waning response to levodopa. Very few PSP patients have a moderate or transient response to dopaminergic agents. This may be because typical PSP patients have little or no limb parkinsonism to begin with, and because there is a widespread involvement of dopaminergic and non-dopaminergic neurotransmitter systems in this disorder. These agents should be tried when patients have parkinsonism, however, as lack of sustained and/or marked benefit from levodopa therapy effectively rules out PD, and helps supports the diagnosis of PSP or other atypical parkinsonism. To evaluate dopaminergic response, we recommend a trial with levodopa–carbidopa up to 1000 mg a day or maximum tolerated dose for at least a month. Dopaminergic agonists are usually less effective but could be tried. PSP patients may develop blepharospasm or retrocollis, and more rarely limb dystonia. In such cases, dopaminergic medication should be cautiously reduced or discontinued to rule out the possibility of treatment-induced dystonia. While PSP patients may develop hallucinations secondary to high doses of medication, hallucinations are not a feature of PSP.

To prevent aspiration, our patient should have a videofluoroscopic modified barium swallow evaluation that could determine if change in food consistency or head position is needed (i.e. thickeners, chin-tuck position). She could also benefit from speech therapy.

A safety inspection of the house by an occupational therapist could prevent the patient from falling, by removing carpets or cluttered furniture. Physical therapy is indicated to improve balance and teach safe transfers. For patients with PSP, we recommend the use of weighted walkers, and physical therapy can train patients how to use them safely. These measures can improve the quality of life and survival of our PSP patients by preventing falls leading to fractures and head injury.

We also refer our patients to an ophthalmologist who can prescribe visual prisms that may help some. Our patient could benefit from using her preserved pursuit to direct her eyes. She should be shown that if she follows her fork she can see the food on her plate. Elevating the plate is also useful. She may benefit from talking books. Natural or artificial tears can treat the keratitis secondary to her severely decreased blinking.

She and her family need to receive education and support to avoid caregiver burden. They can be referred to PSP support groups, if available. It is hoped that in the near future, biological therapies could slow the course of PSP.

Irene Litvan

References

1 Litvan I. Diagnosis and management of progressive supranuclear palsy. *Semin Neurol* 2001; **21**(1): 41–8.
2 Litvan I, Campbell G, Mangone CA *et al.* Which clinical features differentiate progressive supranuclear palsy (Steele–Richardson–Olszewski syndrome) from related disorders? A clinicopathological study. *Brain* 1997; **120**(Pt 1): 65–74.
3 Kaat LD, Boon AJ, Kamphorst W, Ravid R, Duivenvoorden HJ, van Swieten JC. Frontal presentation in progressive supranuclear palsy. *Neurology* 2007; **69**(8): 723–9.
4 Williams DR, de Silva R, Paviour DC *et al.* Characteristics of two distinct clinical phenotypes in pathologically proven progressive supranuclear palsy: Richardson's syndrome and PSP-parkinsonism. *Brain* 2005; **128**(Pt 6): 1247–58.
5 Walter U, Behnke S, Eyding J *et al.* Transcranial brain parenchyma sonography in movement disorders: state of the art. *Ultrasound Med Biol* 2007; **33**(1): 15–25.

Case study 9

Case presentation

A 73-year-old woman with a 7-year history of Parkinson's disease (PD) of the akinetic-rigid type consulted because her motor function had become progressively worse over the past 4 months.

The patient had initially shown a good motor response to a symptomatic treatment with levodopa (in combination with carbidopa) and amantadine. (See Fig. 3.9.1 for doses and medication schedule.) The patient now complained about recurring episodes during which she experienced a marked decline in her motor abilities (so-called "off" time). During these "off" episodes, the patient felt a general stiffness, exhibited a disturbed gait with short shuffled steps and reported difficulties rising from a chair. At first, these motor impairments had only occurred when the patient had forgotten to take the drugs at the usual time. During the preceding months, however, motor function had

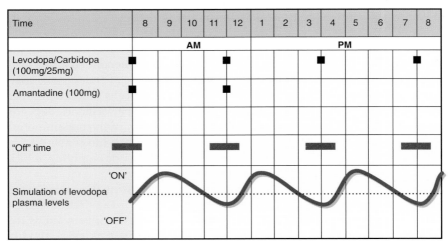

Figure 3.9.1 The relationship between medication, "off" time and levodopa plasma levels.

regularly got worse about 3 h after taking her levodopa medication, and it took up to 1 h after her next dose for motor function to be completely restored. In the morning, it took her at least half an hour after taking her morning medication before she was able to wash and dress.

No painful or involuntary movements were reported. The patient did not show tremor at any time. When we inquired about non-motor symptoms, the patient reported an urge incontinence which got worse during her "off" episodes.

The patient exhibited no psychiatric symptoms such as hallucinations, delusions, or depression. Intellectual abilities were unaltered.

The physical examination was performed in an "on" state 2 h after the patient had taken her drugs. The patient exhibited mild hypomimia and minimal general bradykinesia. Aside from reduced swinging of the left arm and a slightly stooped posture, gait was normal. When we tested rapid alternating movements, the patient exhibited a moderate bradydiadochokinesia on both sides, with the left side being predominantly affected. Slight rigidity was found in the upper and the lower extremities. No dyskinesias or tremor were seen during the examination. The remainder of the neurological examination, including cranial nerve testing, motor function, sensory perception, and coordination, was also unremarkable. Mental status testing revealed no major cognitive deficits. There were no hints of psychiatric disturbances.

Final diagnosis: fluctuations in motor performance: wearing-off.

Discussion

In most patients with early phase PD, symptomatic relief of motor impairments can be achieved with levodopa (in combination with a peripheral L-amino acid decarboxylase (AADC) inhibitor such as benserazide or carbidopa) or a dopamine receptor agonist. Motor abilities are regained owing to the pharmacological substitution of the striatal dopaminergic deficit.

After long-term use of levodopa, however, many PD patients experience motor fluctuations, namely variable levels of motor performance during the course of the day. Several facts account for this phenomenon. First, the neurodegenerative process results in the progressive failure of endogenous compensatory mechanisms, i.e. the number of intact nerve cells that can produce and store dopamine declines and the patient's motor performance depends to a greater extent on the pharmacological substitution of the dopaminergic deficit. Second, levodopa is a short-acting drug with a half-life of about 1.5 h. Third, drug absorption may be impaired by delayed gastric emptying, which is a frequent non-motor symptom in PD patients.

In summary, the variable levels in motor response during the course of the day correlate with the availability of synaptic dopamine in the striatum. When striatal availability of levodopa falls below a certain level (illustrated as the dotted line in Fig. 3.9.1) the typical PD motor symptoms of akinesia, rigidity and tremor emerge.

Autonomic non-motor features of PD (e.g. urge to micturate, sweating, and increased salivation) as well as PD-related psychiatric symptoms (e.g. depressive mood and anxiety) often correlate with "on" and "off" states and thus get worse during "off" episodes [1].

The decline in motor performance between two levodopa doses (with a consecutive recovery between 30 min and 1 h after the next levodopa dose) is termed "wearing-off." Wearing-off presents as relatively predictable "off" episodes with a temporal relationship to the administration of antiparkinsonian drugs. Advanced PD patients can also develop unpredictable "on"/"off" states.

Therapeutic options [2–6]
Adjustment of levodopa dosage
To optimize the continuous striatal availability of the neurotransmitter dopamine, the frequency of levodopa doses can be increased [3]. In the presented patient, we would recommend reducing the temporal window between two levodopa administrations. For example, 100 mg levodopa (in combination with 25 mg carbidopa) could be given every 3 h instead of every 4 h. Thus it should be possible to maintain levodopa above the critical level (i.e. high enough level to ensure a beneficial symptomatic effect).

Addition of a catechol-*O*-methyltransferase (COMT) inhibitor
Peripheral inhibitors of the endogenous dopamine-degrading enzyme COMT are able to stabilize levodopa plasma levels to a certain extent and can, therefore, improve motor fluctuations. At present, two COMT inhibitors are available on the market: entacapone and tolcapone. Tolcapone is clinically superior to entacapone in reducing "off" time, but is potentially hepatotoxic requiring regular liver enzyme monitoring. It is, therefore, considered as a second-line therapy in patients who do not respond to or who cannot tolerate entacapone. Both drugs have shown efficacy in improving wearing-off. In the presented patient, one could add 200 mg entacapone to every levodopa dose. For tolcapone, the standard dosage is 300 mg per day given in three divided doses (3 × 100 mg).

Other therapeutic options
Other therapeutic options to alleviate wearing-off are: (1) addition of a (non-ergot) dopamine receptor agonist; (2) addition of a monoamine oxidase B (MAO-B) inhibitor (e.g. rasagiline 1 mg once a day or selegiline 5 mg once a day); or (3) to switch from standard levodopa formulations to controlled-release (CR) levodopa formulations. In patients who do not respond to these strategies, addition of amantadine can also reduce "off" time. Jejunal levodopa infusion via a portable pump and subcutaneous apomorphine injections represent other high-end therapeutic means for advanced PD patients with motor fluctuations. In severely handicapped patients with an insufficient response to

these therapeutic options (i.e. patients who still exhibit marked motor fluctuations (and dyskinesias)), deep brain stimulation should be considered.

Soluble levodopa formulations (which act faster than the standard levodopa formulations) can be used to treat early morning akinesia. CR levodopa formulations at night can reduce nocturnal akinesia.

The goal of the therapeutic options discussed above is to enhance dopaminergic stimulation in the striatum. As an untoward side effect, however, these can induce or worsen dyskinesias.

It seems reasonable to switch from standard levodopa to CR levodopa formulations to treat wearing-off. This approach, however, is not always successful due to the variable levels of absorption of levodopa (see above).

Dietary proteins hamper the absorption of levodopa in the small intestine, thereby decreasing levodopa levels, and consequently can provoke or worsen motor fluctuations. Hence, PD patients should be instructed to take their levodopa doses 1 h prior to or 1 h after a (protein-rich) meal.

Marcus M. Unger, Wolfgang H. Oertel

References

1 Quinn NP. Classification of fluctuations in patients with Parkinson's disease. *Neurology* 1998; **51**(2 Suppl 2): S25–9.

2 Horstink M, Tolosa E, Bonuccelli U *et al.*; European Federation of Neurological Societies; Movement Disorder Society-European Section. Review of the therapeutic management of Parkinson's disease. Report of a joint task force of the European Federation of Neurological Societies (EFNS) and the Movement Disorder Society-European Section (MDS-ES). Part II: late (complicated) Parkinson's disease. *Eur J Neurol* 2006; **13**(11): 1186–202.

3 Rascol O, Brooks DJ, Melamed E *et al.*; LARGO study group. Rasagiline as an adjunct to levodopa in patients with Parkinson's disease and motor fluctuations (LARGO, Lasting effect in Adjunct therapy with Rasagiline Given Once daily, study): a randomised, double-blind, parallel-group trial. *Lancet* 2005; **365**(9463): 947–54.

4 Brooks DJ, Agid Y, Eggert K, Widner H, Ostergaard K, Holopainen A; TC-INIT Study Group. Treatment of end-of-dose wearing-off in Parkinson's disease: stalevo (levodopa/carbidopa/entacapone) and levodopa/DDCI given in combination with Comtess/Comtan (entacapone) provide equivalent improvements in symptom control superior to that of traditional levodopa/DDCI treatment. *Eur Neurol* 2005; **53**(4): 197–202.

5 Adler CH, Singer C, O'Brien C *et al.* Randomized, placebo-controlled study of tolcapone in patients with fluctuating Parkinson disease treated with levodopa-carbidopa. Tolcapone Fluctuator Study Group III. *Arch Neurol* 1998; **55**(8): 1089–95.

6 Ahlskog JE, Muenter MD, McManis PG, Bell GN, Bailey PA. Controlled-release Sinemet (CR-4): a double-blind crossover study in patients with fluctuating Parkinson's disease. *Mayo Clin Proc* 1988; **63**(9): 876–86.

Case study 10

Case presentation

Mrs CB developed Parkinson's disease (PD) when she was 41 years old. On the first examination, she had resting tremor on the left hand, mild bradykinesia and muscular rigidity on the same side. Gait and postural stability were normal. She had no family history for neurological diseases and she had not been exposed to drugs or toxins. She was put on a dopamine agonist with good response. When levodopa was added about 4 years later, she was taking 4.5 mg of pramipexole plus 3 mg of cabergoline – a strategy used to prolong dopamine agonist monotherapy. She was now generally slow, her left hand was not functioning properly and she also had signs on the right-hand side. She responded well to levodopa, Sinemet 100/25 q.i.d. However, about 2 years later, she started to complain about "strange movements and cramps in the left foot" which appeared around lunch time and lasted for about 15–20 min.

On examination, her parkinsonism was well controlled but she showed mild dyskinesias of the trunk and head of which she was not aware. Cabergoline was decreased to 2 mg/day and withdrawn after 2 months because of the persistence of abnormal movements. In the mean time, she was still complaining about the movement of her left foot.

After a few more months, the movements became more severe and painful and involved also the left arm and leg. She was hospitalized for observation. On taking the morning dose of levodopa and pramipexole, her parkinsonism was very well controlled; she only had mild bradykinesia in her left hand, but otherwise was normal. There were no dyskinesias during the morning. At 12.15 hours, after the second dose of levodopa and pramipexole, she started to develop painful dystonia of the foot and choreic movement of the left arm and leg. She was unable to walk or perform any tasks with her left side, whereas on the right she just became more bradykinetic. After 30 min, these symptoms disappeared and her condition returned to normal. At this point a genetic study was performed which did not show any of the then-known mutations.

Pramipexole was reduced to 3 mg/day; but the movements persisted and were followed by 1 h of akinesia and rigidity ("off" period). At this point pramipexole was increased back to 4.5 mg/day and levodopa increased to 100/25 five times (3-h intervals).

The patient remained well controlled on this regime for a few years, but occasionally she had periods of severe choreic/dystonic movement during the day and in the evening. Mild choreic dyskinesias were present continuously.

Some time later, the crises reappeared but were now very severe, involving the whole body but especially the legs. These always started in the left foot. During the crises, the patient looked like an out-of-control marionette. The crises were always followed by profound "off" periods. To find the correlation with levodopa levels, concentrations in the blood were measured and revealed that the crises followed the decrease of levodopa levels and finished when the level was close to zero. It was clear that the patient was suffering from severe diphasic dyskinesias.

Different strategies were tried, including the administration of a catechol-O-methyltransferase (COMT) inhibitor and anticholinergics, but to no avail. The injection of apomorphine by penject did stop the movements, but very often they reappeared 45–60 min later. Apomorphine infusion was successful but had to be discontinued after a few months because of psychiatric side effects.

Eventually, intrajejunal levodopa infusion was given. The abnormal movements disappeared during the day but were always present at the end of the day when the pump was turned off. After some months, the abnormal movements appeared after 10 h of infusion despite the pump being on. Analysis showed that the movement started when the plasma levodopa concentration was still at the usual constant level and disappeared once the pump was turned off when levodopa was close to zero (Fig. 3.10.1).

Today the patient is on 10 h continuous levodopa infusion and has 15–20 min of abnormal movement before the pump is switched off.

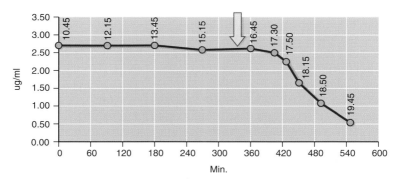

Figure 3.10.1 Levodopa plasma level during intrajejunal infusion of levodopa. Arrow, the time when the dyskinesias started. Dyskinesias disappeared at 19.45 hours when the levodopa level was close to zero.

Differential diagnosis

Abnormal involuntary movements (AIMs) are a commonly observed side effect in chronically levodopa-treated PD patients [1]. AIMs in fluctuating parkinsonian patients may be classified on the basis of their course and clinical phenomenology following a regular or over-threshold dose of oral levodopa. In this respect the most common forms of AIMs are off-period dystonias, diphasic dyskinesias (onset- and end-of-dose dyskinesias), and peak-dose dyskinesias.

"Off"-period dystonia is generally correlated to the akinesia which precedes the full effect of levodopa. It mainly involves the foot on the more affected side and includes painful toe extension [2]. It can also appear in the morning before the first levodopa intake (early morning dystonia). It is generally assumed that onset- and end-of-dose dyskinesias correlate respectively with the rise and fall of plasma levodopa levels, while peak-dose (or benefit-of-dose) dyskinesias correlate with plateau plasma levodopa levels. Peak-dose dyskinesias are typically choreiform, but may manifest as dystonia, myoclonus, or other movement disorders. They are most prominent in the head, face, neck, trunk, and upper extremities. The less common diphasic dyskinesias [3,4] consist of repetitive, alternating, asymmetric, stereotypic movements that primarily involve the lower extremities [5–7]. In contrast to peak-dose dyskinesia, diphasic dyskinesias are associated with relatively low plasma levodopa levels and characteristically disappear with higher or lower plasma levodopa concentrations. Diphasic dyskinesias are frequently observed in conjunction with parkinsonian features in other body regions [8].

AIMs commonly appear first in the foot, ipsilaterally to the most affected parkinsonian side of the body, with inversion of the foot and ankle. This finding is explained by the early loss of dopaminergic innervation in the dorsolateral striatum, which corresponds somatotopically to the foot area innervated by the substantia nigra [9]. Later in the course of the disease, dyskinesias may spread to other areas of the body. This pattern may follow the same pattern of progression of parkinsonian symptoms. The various forms of dyskinesias are not mutually exclusive, and combination of choreic and dystonic movements, and peak-dose and end-of-dose dyskinesias often occur in the same patient.

Most of the time, patients are not aware of mild benefit-of-dose dyskinesias and usually they do not complain about them. In contrast, patients always complain about diphasic dyskinesias, which are very distressing, sometimes painful, and accompanied by periods of limited mobility. They usually appear when levodopa starts to produce its effect and when levodopa wears off, but they can also be present during only one of the two phases. Usually, end-of-dose dyskinesias are more prolonged than those at onset of dose and more disabling for the patient.

Our patient was suffering from mild peak-dose dyskinesias but also from severe diphasic dyskinesias that sometimes appeared during the day and, most often, in the evening. Once she was treated with continuous intrajejunal levodopa infusion, peak-dose dyskinesias disappeared, but diphasic dyskinesias persisted, especially at the end of the day. Movements were primarily comprised of asymmetric, rhythmic, alternating, stereotypic movements that predominantly affected the leg [4,7]. Dyskinesias in our patient occurred in association with incomplete improvement in parkinsonian status. We have observed similar dyskinesias to those we report here during continuous infusion of dopaminergic therapies associated with periods of incomplete motor improvement. These patients experienced prolonged periods of repetitive, stereotypic, dyskinetic movements of the legs accompanied by parkinsonism in other body regions that subsided with increases in the infusion rate or by ending the infusion [10].

Final diagnosis: mild peak-dose and severe diphasic dyskinesias.

Discussion

The pathophysiology of diphasic dyskinesias is not clear; however, the observation that these movements appear when levodopa reaches a threshold above which the patient turns "on" leads to the hypothesis that they are the consequence of suboptimal stimulation of the dopaminergic system. Diphasic dyskinesias can be very long if the level of levodopa remains at the threshold level such as during a suboptimal dose during an infusion or during treatment with slow-release preparations of levodopa.

In some cases (such as the one reported here), diphasic dyskinesias may appear even if the plasma levodopa level is sufficiently high. This could be owing to a saturation of the system with a consequent dopaminergic hypostimulation. They could also represent a phenomenon owing to tolerance caused by continuous infusion which, instead of producing immediate "off" periods, produces diphasic dyskinesias followed by the "off" period. This hypothesis may be supported by the fact that the patient becomes a responder again the day after a drug-free night.

A severe form of dyskinesias similar to those observed in our patient has been reported in PD patients who have undergone fetal nigral transplantation [11–13]. These dyskinesias persisted following complete withdrawal of dopaminergic medication and were defined as "off-medication dyskinesias." This contrasts with classical levodopa-induced dyskinesias (either peak-dose or diphasic), which typically disappear after stopping the drug. The authors formulate the hypothesis that these dyskinesias, phenomenologically similar to diphasic dyskinesias, may reflect partial but inadequate graft survival that is sufficient to produce, store, and release low doses of dopamine for a prolonged period after a dose of levodopa, but insufficient to induce an antiparkinsonian response [13].

Treatment

Treatment of dyskinesias in general remains difficult and is sometimes frustrating for patients and physicians. Diphasic dyskinesias are even more difficult to manage. Prolonged-release preparations of levodopa should be substituted with an immediate-release formula to avoid the prolongation of end-of-dose dyskinesias. Amantadine and sometimes anticholinergics, especially if dystonias are present, can be helpful. In some patients, apomorphine penject can be efficacious. Continuous apomorphine subcutaneous infusion is effective in most patients; continuous levodopa intrajejunal infusion controls dyskinesias during the day but in some patients end-of-dose dyskinesias appear when levodopa is discontinued.

Fabrizio Stocchi

References

1 Fahn S. The spectrum of levodopa-induced dyskinesias. *Ann Neurol* 2000; **47**(Suppl 1): 2–11.

2 Vidailhet M, Bonnet AM, Marconi R. The phenomenology of L-dopa-induced dyskinesias in Parkinson's disease. *Mov Disord* 1999; **14**(Suppl 1): 13–18.

3 Lhermitte F, Agid Y, Signoret JL, Studler JM. Les dyskinésies de "début et fin de dose" provoquées par la L-DOPA. *Rev Neurol* (Paris)1977; **133**: 297–308.

4 Muenter MD, Sharpless NS, Tyce GM, Darley FL. Patterns of dystonia ("I-D-I" and "D-I-D-") in response to L-dopa therapy for Parkinson's disease. *Mayo Clin Proc* 1977; **52**: 163–74.

5 Luquin MR, Scipioni O, Vaamonde J, Gershanik O, Obeso JA. Levodopa-induced dyskinesias in Parkinson's disease: clinical and pharmacological classification. *Mov Disord* 1992; **7**: 117–22.

6 De Saint Victor JF, Pollak P, Gervason CL, Perret J. Levodopa-induced diphasic dyskinesias improved by subcutaneous apomorphine. *Mov Disord* 1992; **7**: 283–4.

7 Marconi R, Lefebre-Caparros D, Bonnet AM, Vidailhet M, Dubois B, Agid Y. Levodopa-induced dyskinesias in Parkinson's disease: phenomenology and pathophysiology. *Mov Disord* 1994; **9**: 2–12.

8 Fahn S. Fluctuations of disability in Parkinson's disease: pathophysiology. In: Marsden CD, Fahn S, eds. *Movement Disorders 2*. London, UK: Butterworth Scientific, 1981: 123–45.

9 Fearnley JM, Lees AJ. Ageing and Parkinson's disease: substantia nigra regional selectivity. *Brain* 1991; **9**: 2–12.

10 Stocchi F, Vacca L, Ruggieri S, Olanow CW. Intermittent vs continuous levodopa administration in patients with advanced Parkinson disease: a clinical and pharmacokinetic study. *Arch Neurol* 2005; **62**(6): 905–10.

11 Freed CR, Greene PE, Breeze RE *et al*. Transplantation of embryonic dopamine neurons for severe Parkinson's disease. *N Engl J Med* 2001; **344**: 710–19.

12 Hagell P, Piccini P, Bjorklund A *et al*. Dyskinesias following neural transplantation in Parkinson's disease. *Nat Neurosci* 2002; **5**: 627–8.

13 Olanow CW, Goetz CG, Kordower JH *et al*. A double blind placebo-controlled trial of bilateral fetal nigral transplantation in Parkinson's disease. *Ann Neurol* 2003; **54**: 403–14.

Case presentation

A 54-year-old right-handed aeronautical engineer suffering from Parkinson's disease (PD) was admitted to the hospital because of a 6-month history of increasingly severe evening attacks of abnormal lower-limb movements and chest pain.

PD had been diagnosed 7 years before, after the patient complained of right-hand clumsiness and micrographia. The initial treatment consisted of a dopamine agonist to which levodopa was added 2 years later. During this time, the functional impact of the disease was mild, enabling the patient to maintain his professional activities. However, 1 year before admission he began to suffer from disabling PD symptoms, which generally occurred 3–3.5 h after taking levodopa. He also reported painful contraction of the right leg and extension of the big toe in the morning, a few minutes after awakening.

During the 6 months prior to admission, his neurological status progressively worsened and he was obliged to stop working. This period was marked by attacks of abnormal movements. The attacks usually started between 6:00 and 6:30 PM and lasted until about 9:00 PM, whereupon he returned to his usual state. The abnormal movements consisted of repetitive violent "pedaling" movements of the legs and were sometimes associated with intermittent contraction of the right upper limb with sustained hyperextension of the arm and flexion of the fingers. Profuse sweating (the patient had to change his shirt at least once), tachycardia, anxiety, and constrictive chest pain accompanied these movements. He was able to walk almost normally, but experienced difficulty in writing or using a computer keyboard. Following an attack, the patient was exhausted.

The attacks worsened in severity and duration after the patient's neurologist decreased his afternoon levodopa intake by 50 mg. During the 6 months before admission, the patient lost 6 kg in weight. He had no known health problems other than PD and no risk factors for vascular disease. Treatment at

Table 3.11.1 Patient's daily treatment at time of admission

Time of intake	8:00 AM	12:00 AM	4:00 PM	8:00 PM	Total
Ropinirole (mg)	3	3	3	3	12
L-DOPA (mg)	150	150	100[a]	150	550

[a] Reduced from 150 mg four weeks before admission.

admission was ropinirole 12 mg/day and levodopa 550 mg/day, in four doses (Table 3.11.1).

On examination (10:30 AM), the patient appeared tired but considered himself to be in a "good state." He made abrupt, brief movements of the head, which were accentuated while speaking. The patient claimed not to be really aware of these movements, but explained that his wife had noticed them for about 1 year. The right side of his body was slightly akinetic, as evidenced by irregularities during alternate thumb-to-index tapping, hand closing and opening, and foot tapping. There was no PD rigidity and muscle tone was low. The remainder of the examination was normal.

Differential diagnosis

Our patient had a 7-year history of idiopathic PD. The good and sustained response to dopaminergic drugs, as attested by the paucity of residual PD symptoms during the examination 2.5 h after drug intake, and the absence of other neurological symptoms or signs supported the diagnosis. His attacks had started about 6 months after he had begun to suffer from motor fluctuations (i.e. fluctuations occurring when the beneficial effects of the treatment wore off prior to the next dose). The attacks consisted of chest pain in conjunction with dysautonomic symptoms (sweating, tachycardia, anxiety) and abnormal movements.

Intercurrent medical conditions. The patient reported symptoms compatible with attacks of angina pectoris: constrictive chest pain and dysautonomic symptoms. They were not induced by physical exercise, though the severe movements that he complained of might be considered as an equivalent. The patient did not, however, report any similar pain during other physical activities. Furthermore, the attacks lasted for over 3 h, which would be unusual for angina pectoris, and he had no special risk factor for coronary artery disease. An electrocardiogram during an attack would help to verify this point.

Drug-induced dyskinesias. The development of intermittent abnormal movements in a PD patient after several years of levodopa treatment, especially when motor fluctuations have occurred, strongly suggests the diagnosis of levodopa-induced dyskinesias (LID). There are three main types of LID: "off"-period dystonia, peak-dose dyskinesias, and diphasic dyskinesias [1] (see Figure 3.11.1). What type of LID was this patient suffering from during the evening attacks?

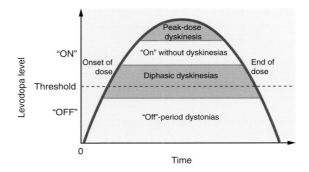

Figure 3.11.1

"Off"-period dystonia. As suggested by the name, such LIDs present as dystonia, i.e. a sustained muscle contraction leading to repetitive torsion movements or abnormal posture, and accompanying a period of recurrence of PD symptoms ("off" state). Typically, it is localized in the foot on the more severely affected side, is usually observed a few minutes after awakening, and disappears when the treatment starts to improve PD symptoms. This patient reported this type of LID in the morning. The abnormal movements he experienced during the evening attacks, however, were different; they were not exclusively dystonic and were not concomitant with severe parkinsonism ("off" state).

Peak-dose dyskinesias. These are the most common type of LID and are mainly choreic, preferentially affecting the upper limbs, head and trunk. Muscle tone is low and the patient is more or less unaware of such movements. They are also typically reinforced during motor or mental tasks. Furthermore, they are observed when dopaminergic drugs exert their maximal beneficial effect (best "on" state). This patient presented such movements during the neurological examination. These dyskinesias, which did not cause the patient any distress and were present at a time when he was greatly improved by the treatment were, however, different from the abnormal movements accompanying the evening attacks.

Diphasic dyskinesias (onset-of-dose and end-of-dose dyskinesias). In contrast to peak-dose dyskinesias, these LIDs usually predominate in the lower limbs and tend to be ballistic or dystonic. Some repetitive "pedaling" limb movements have been reported. The abnormal movements presented by the patient during the evening attacks are thus highly suggestive of diphasic dyskinesias. As in this observation, diphasic dyskinesias are often distressing and can be accompanied by anxiety, tachycardia, thoracic oppression, and chest or abdominal pain. They correlate with the rise and fall of the beneficial effects of the dopaminergic drug. In this observation, the dyskinesias were probably concomitant with the decreasing beneficial effects of the 4:00 PM drug intake, thus corresponding to end-of-dose dyskinesias. The patient reported some difficulty in writing or working with a keyboard, indicating a probable intermediate level of correction of parkinsonism. Moreover, the dyskinesias stopped one hour after the 8:00 PM drug intake, when the treatment attained a level able to correct PD symptoms. The worsening of the attacks induced by the decrease in the dosage of the 4:00 PM drug intake was fully compatible with the diagnosis. Given that this type of LID is concomitant with a level of dopaminergic correction just below that at which PD symptoms are fully improved, it is not surprising that such dyskinesias have been shown to be improved – at least in the short term – by increasing the dosage of levodopa (Table 3.11.2) [2].

Final diagnosis: end-of-dose dyskinesia.

Discussion

Diphasic dyskinesias occur in 15–20% of patients chronically treated with levodopa. They are less well known than the more frequent peak-dose dys-kinesias. It is important to differentiate between these two types of LID, as they are treated differently. Schematically, peak-dose dyskinesias and dipha-sic dyskinesias can be contrasted point by point in terms of time of occur-rence after drug intake, concomitant parkinsonian state, type of abnormal movement, and body localization (Table 3.11.2). Differentiating between them, however, can sometimes be challenging. Even with the help of the caregiver, the patient is not always able to accurately describe the time of occurrence and the type of movements. Moreover, in some patients there is a continuum between onset-of-dose, peak-dose, and end-of-dose dyskinesias. There may also be rapid oscillations between the two types of dyskinesias, which may even coexist in different segments of the body [3]. Clinical observation of the patient during a full day (during hospitalization or by specialized nurses at the patient's home) or a levodopa challenge can be an invaluable source of information in such cases.

The management of LID is one of the most difficult problems in the treat-ment of PD, and among the different forms of LID, diphasic dyskinesias are probably the hardest to improve. It must, however, be acknowledged that there have not been many trials to assess strategies for reducing LID and hardly any have specifically analyzed the effect on the different types of LID. The fol-lowing proposals are thus mainly based on the views of experts in published review articles [1], and on our own clinical practice.

The first step in LID treatment is to try to modify the antiparkinsonian medication. In contrast to peak-dose dyskinesias, for which the usual treat-ment is to decrease the individual dose of levodopa immediately preceeding the dyskinesias (at the risk of worsening wearing-off phenomena), diphasic dyskinesias require the antiparkinsonian treatment to be slightly increased. Increasing levodopa dosage before the period of diphasic dyskinesias usually improves them [2]. The beneficial effects of this strategy are limited in time, however, and the diphasic dyskinesias re-emerge with greater severity a few

Table 3.11.2 Principal characteristics of the three main types of dyskinesias

	'Off'-period dystonia	Peak-dose dyskinesias	Diphasic dyskinesias; onset-of-dose dyskinesias (ODD) and end-of-dose dyskinesias (EDD)
Timing	Early morning	~ 1–3 h after L-dopa intake (at a phase during which PD symptoms are clearly improved)	Shortly after ODD and before EDD L-dopa intake (typically after ODD or before EDD phase of parkinsonism)
Parkinsonian symptoms	Severe	Minimal	Intermediate
Muscle tone	PD rigidity + dystonia	Hypotonia	Mild to moderate PD rigidity ± dystonia
Predominant type of dyskinesias	Dystonia	Chorea	Dystonia Ballism Myoclonus Repetitive movements
Preferential body localization	Foot	Head, trunk, upper limbs	Lower limbs

weeks after such treatment. A better option is to try to increase the dosage of a dopamine agonist with a subsequent decrease in the individual levodopa dosage should peak-dose dyskinesias appear. In other words, the treatment should tend towards an almost "non-pulsatile" brain dopaminergic correction. In that way, hourly or even half-hourly administration of very low doses of liquid levodopa, subcutaneous apomorphine infusion, or intraduodenal infusion of levodopa gel may help some patients.

In a second step, some drugs such as amantadine or clozapine used as add-on treatment could have some antidyskinetic activity, and thus may also lead to beneficial effects on diphasic dyskinesias, although this has not yet been clearly demonstrated. Stereotactic surgery (pallidotomy, deep brain stimulation (DBS) applied to the globus pallidus or to the subthalamic nucleus) reduces LIDs, including diphasic dyskinesias, as has been clearly demonstrated in the case of subthalamic DBS [4]. Such a therapeutic option could be considered in the most severe cases.

Philippe Damier

References

1 Fabbrini G, Brotchie JM, Grandas F, Nomoto M, Goetz CG. Levodopa-induced dyskinesias. *Mov Disord* 2007; **22**: 1379–89.
2 Lhermitte F, Agid Y, Signoret JL. Onset and end-of-dose dyskinesias. *Arch Neurol* 1978; **35**: 261–2.
3 Marconi R, Lefebvre-Caparros D, Bonnet AM, Vidailhet M, Dubois B, Agid Y. Levodopa-induced dyskinesias in Parkinson's disease: phenomenology and pathophysiology. *Mov Disord* 1994; **9**: 2–12.
4 Deuschl G, Shade-Brittinger C, Krack P *et al*. A randomized trial of deep-brain stimulation for Parkinson's disease. *N Engl J Med* 2006; **355**: 896–908.

Case presentation

Ms M., a 74-year-old white female was admitted to our clinic because she was no longer able to successfully carry out activities of daily living. In the morning she was unable to get up and prepare her breakfast. She had told her physician that she had difficulties concentrating and remembering, felt increasingly empty and hopeless, was tired of living, and had almost totally withdrawn from her relatives and friends.

Ms M. had been diagnosed with Parkinson's disease (PD) 3 years previously by her neurologist, on presenting with gait instability followed by right-sided rigidity and akinesia. These motor symptoms were well controlled by treatment with levodopa (425 mg per day). Around 2 years later, Ms M. gradually developed depressive symptoms including reduced appetite and weight loss, physical and social anhedonia, terminal insomnia, and the feeling of inner emptiness. Her motor symptoms, however, did not change. She had been treated by her physician with amitriptyline (100 mg per day) over a period of 6 weeks before being admitted to our clinic because of suicidal ideation in addition to her other symptoms. During her consultation with us, she related that these symptoms had worsened during the last 2 weeks. She had very little appetite and had lost almost 8 kg during the last 6 months. She was unable to sleep through the night and usually woke up early in the morning without being able to go back to sleep.

Ms M. recalled that she had experienced episodes of lowered mood earlier in her life, mostly during fall and winter, whereas during the summer she had experienced periods of happiness, elevated mood, and an increased level of activities. She had never, however, seen a doctor about these mood swings. In general, she described herself as a socially active person, who liked to travel and was normally very interested in what was going on around her. About 8 years previously, she had consulted her general practitioner because she suffered from depressed mood and lack of drive and was treated with St John's wort (*Hypericum perforatum*) for 6 months until symptoms remitted.

Differential diagnosis and treatment

On Ms M.'s admission to our clinic, laboratory tests including thyroid-stimulating hormone, blood glucose, glycosylated hemoglobin (Hb_{A1c}), and cell counts, as well as an electrocardiogram (ECG) and an electroencephalograph (EEG), did not show any pathological alterations. Initially, she was treated with lorazepam (1 mg/day) and supportive psychotherapy because of suicidal ideation. Thoughts about committing suicide were no longer present after 2 days of inpatient treatment. Amitriptyline was tapered because of lack of antidepressant efficacy and intolerable side effects including constipation and impaired cognition. Subsequently, side effects related to anticholinergic mechanisms including constipation declined.

While reducing the amitriptyline, levodopa was kept at a stable dosage and treatment with fluoxetine (20 mg/day) was initiated. After 2 weeks, fluoxetine was increased to 40 mg/day because mood, cognitive functions, and sleep improved only mildly. Despite antidepressant medication, 4 weeks later Ms M. was still suffering from depressive symptoms including reduced appetite, anhedonia, loss of interest, lack of drive, social withdrawal, and inability to perform her daily activities. Cognitive impairment, however, had disappeared. On the other hand, right dominating rigidity and cogwheel phenomena in upper and lower extremities had increased. Therefore, fluoxetine was stopped. Motor phenomena including rigidity declined, but did not fully disappear.

Brain magnetic resonance imaging, conducted to exclude structural changes that could cause the persistent symptoms of depression, did not show any signs of atrophy or other significant pathological alterations.

Given that dopamine agonists are well tolerated in patients of higher age as shown in large study populations during treatment in clinical practice, the dopamine agonist pramipexole was started with a daily dosage of 0.35 mg gradually increased to 2.1 mg over 3 weeks. Dosage of levodopa was not altered. Initially, zolpidem was prescribed for sleep disturbances. Transient nausea, sweating, and feelings of slight agitation disappeared after 2 weeks. Ms M. developed more interest in her surroundings and in contact with her caregivers. Appetite increased and Ms M. reported actually enjoying her meals for the first time since the onset of depression. In addition, motor function improved. There were no side effects on gastrointestinal functions or motor performance, and no changes in blood count, ECG, or EEG.

After release from the hospital, pramipexole (2.1 mg/day) and levodopa (425 mg/day) were continued at stable dosages. Three months later, Ms M was socially active again and able to perform her daily activities.

Final diagnosis: PD-related depression.

Discussion

The case presented shows that depressive symptoms in PD need to be carefully evaluated. Depression is the most frequent neuropsychiatric complication in

PD, affecting about 40–50% of all patients. It reduces quality of life independent of motor symptoms, may manifest as one of the first symptoms of PD, and seems to be underrated and undertreated [1,2]. The diagnosis is complicated because clinical symptoms of depression may overlap with or be mistaken for those of PD, including flattening of affect, psychomotor retardation, sleep disturbances, loss of desire, and anhedonia [3]. Depressive syndromes in patients with PD qualitatively differ from primary major depression. Guilt, sense of failure, self blame, suicide, but not suicidal ideation, are less frequent [4]. One ongoing European multicenter study, Profile of Depressive Symptoms in PD (PRODEST-PD), has been designed to identify the relationship between the cognitive, mood, and motor symptoms of PD and patient scores on depression rating scales in a naturalistic setting [5].

Anxiety and depressive symptoms are not only associated with PD, but may be the first manifestation of PD years before the onset of motor symptoms [6]. Patients suffering from major depression seem to be at a higher risk of developing PD. Depressive episodes, as demonstrated by the patient presented, may be part of the early progression of PD and it is unknown whether adequate and rigorous treatment of depression may lower the risk of developing PD later on.

Depression is not purely a reaction to neurological deficits in PD and there is no linear relationship between severity of depression and dopamine deficiency caused by PD [1,4]. Ms M.'s depression was associated with rigidity, bradykinesia, and postural gait disturbances. The finding may indicate that depression is more likely associated with PD symptoms that are responsive to treatment with dopaminergic medication. In addition, experimental and clinical studies indicate non-dopaminergic cerebral lesions in PD that might explain depressive symptoms, for instance affecting brain stem nuclei including the raphe nucleus and corresponding serotonergic projections, or the locus coeruleus and noradrenergic pathways [7].

Tri- and tetracyclic antidepressants (TCAs) such as amitriptyline have been the most commonly used antidepressants in depressed patients with PD. Only five randomized, controlled, double-blind studies exist concerning the efficacy of TCAs in PD [1]. The use of TCAs in elderly patients is restricted by their anticholinergic effects, which may improve motor functions but worsen cognition. Selective serotonin reuptake inhibitors (SSRI) have a similar efficacy to TCAs, but show a different profile of adverse effects, and thus may perhaps be preferable in elderly patients [1]. There is, however, a lack of controlled studies in patients with PD and depression. Worsening of PD motor symptoms in the reported case may be the result of treatment with fluoxetine. This has been indicated by single case reports before, but reported as a rare phenomenon in larger retrospective studies [8]. Motor symptoms such as rigidity, tremor, and akinesia are particularly prone to worsening during treatment with SSRIs and should be monitored carefully in the individual patient.

Experimental findings indicate anxiolytic properties for ropinirole and antidepressant and anti-anhedonic effects for pramipexole, which may be related to its specific action on D_3/D_2 receptors in mesolimbic and prefrontal cortical projections [9]. In addition, clinical studies show antidepressant effects of dopamine agonists in patients with major and bipolar depression. Open and controlled studies in depressed patients with PD show therapeutic effects of pramipexole on motor functions, depressed mood and anhedonia and possibly antidepressant effects of ropinirole. Randomized controlled data show at least comparable effects between the SSRI sertraline and pramipexole [10]. In addition, dopamine agonists are regarded as a well-tolerated and safe treatment alternative in elderly patients, as has been shown in large observational studies [11]. To avoid multiple drug interactions and possible side effects of antidepressants, patients with PD and depression may benefit from a global therapeutic approach with dopamine agonists improving both motor and depressive symptoms [1].

Matthias R. Lemke

References

1 Lemke MR, Fuchs G, Gemende I et al. Depression and Parkinson's disease. J Neurol 2004; **251**(S6): VI/24–7.
2 Richard IH, Kurlan R. A survey of antidepressant drug use in Parkinson's disease. Parkinson Study Group. Neurology 1997; **49**: 1168–70.
3 Allain H, Schuck S, Mauduit N. Depression in Parkinson's disease. BMJ 2000; **320**: 1287–8.
4 Cummings JL. Depression and Parkinson's disease: a review. Am J Psychiatry 1992; **149**: 443–54.
5 Barone P, Groot AA de, Goetz CG et al. Depressive symptoms in Parkinson's disease: design and methods of a prospective observational study. Mov Disord 2006; **21**(Suppl 15): P548 (abstract).
6 Shiba M, Bower JH, Maraganore DM et al. Anxiety disorders and depressive disorders preceding Parkinson's disease: a case-control study. Mov Disord 2000; **15**: 669–77.
7 Mayberg HS, Solomon DH. Depression in Parkinson's disease: a biochemical and organic viewpoint. Adv Neurol 1995; **65**: 49–60.
8 Richard IH, Maughn A, Kurlan R. Do serotonin reuptake inhibitor antidepressants worsen Parkinson's disease? A retrospective case series. Mov Disord 1999; **14**: 155–7.
9 Lemke MR. Antidepressant effects of dopamine agonists: experimental and clinical findings. Nervenarzt 2007; **78**: 31–8.
10 Barone P, Scarzella L, Marconi R et al.; Depression/Parkinson Italian Study Group. Pramipexole versus sertraline in the treatment of depression in Parkinson's disease: a national multicenter parallel-group randomized study. J Neurol 2006; **253**: 601–7.
11 Lemke MR, Brecht HM, Koester J, Kraus PH, Reichmann H. Anhedonia, depression, and motor functioning in Parkinson's disease during treatment with pramipexole. J Neuropsychiat Clin Neurosci 2005; **17**: 214–20.

Case study 13

Case presentation

A 56-year-old right-handed university professor of physics was admitted to the movement disorders unit to evaluate the possibility of deep brain stimulation (DBS) for his Parkinson's disease (PD).

The patient had been in excellent health until the age of 46, when fatigue, micrographia, and decrease in right arm swing while walking developed. PD diagnosis was made 4 months later when a small-amplitude rest tremor of the right fingers appeared. This patient had no noteworthy medical or surgical history except that his systolic blood pressure was often 150 mmHg. The patient's father had had dementia (possibly Alzheimer's disease) and had died at the age of 85. Pergolide was given at increasing doses up to 4.5 mg/day with major benefit on all parkinsonian symptoms. Two years later, levodopa/carbidopa was introduced because hand tremor was not well controlled.

The "honeymoon" period ended 3 years later with the appearance of end-of-dose akinesia, tremor, and inverted dystonic posture of the right foot. "On"-period mild repetitive dyskinesias of the neck and right leg were observed but not noticed by the patient. Entacapone was associated with levodopa/carbidopa, which was divided into five daily doses of 150 mg each every 3 h. Over the course of the next 4 years, "on" dyskinesias became disabling and he also suffered from motor fluctuations with shuffling gait and painful akinetic-rigid right hemibody during "off" periods that could last 2 h by the end of the afternoon. The patient had to stop working. He divorced his wife who complained because he had become irritable, suspicious, and jealous. She reported that her husband spent almost all night long on his computer visiting pornographic websites. Pergolide was switched to ropinirole 18 mg/day and the daily dose was progressively decreased to 6 mg/day to control the behavioral, psychotic, and impulse control disorders. In parallel, all levodopa-induced motor complications worsened and periods of severe akinesia appeared, hindering walking. The patient spent a mean total of 4 h/day with severe gait impairment associated with freezing, but no falls. Apomorphine injections were effective for these periods. Getting up from bed at night was extremely difficult and leg pain became a major complaint. Brain imaging had not been done. One year before admission, a trial of apomorphine infusion was carried out but was discontinued after a few months because of the persistence of disabling biphasic dyskinesias. The patient was, therefore, sent by his neurologist to a center specializing in the surgical treatment of PD by DBS.

Physical examination showed general good health, and normal total body mass and vital signs. The blood pressure during on-motor periods was 140/80 mmHg. Neurological examination revealed an alert, oriented, attentive man; however, he had difficulties providing the details of his pharmacological history. He scored 28 out of 30 on the Mini Mental State Examination, and 15 out of 18 on the Frontal Assessment Battery (2 out of 3 on the verbal fluency, motor sequence and go/no-go task items). At the time of the examination during which he was under the effect of levodopa, his speech was moderately dysarthric and hypophonic. He did not hallucinate or communicate paranoid ideas and had no delusions. His mood appeared normal and he was very enthusiastic about surgical treatment with the main expectation to be able to walk normally and speak around the clock. He had moderate chronic constipation and frequent urinary emergencies, but no incontinence.

Neurological examination was normal, except for the signs and symptoms related to PD. During the examination, his entire body was affected by repetitive choreic dystonic movements with a clear predominance on the right and in his neck. No tremor or rigidity was noticed.

The ability to make rapid, alternating movements was mildly reduced in the right arm, mainly because of the abnormal involuntary movements. He rose easily from a chair, walked normally, and his postural stability was almost normal as assessed by the pull test.

Magnetic resonance imaging (MRI) showed mild cortical atrophy and some hyperintensities in the white matter on T2-weighted sequences. Routine laboratory test results including blood coagulation were normal. Chest X-ray and electrocardiogram were normal.

Discussion

Age

This patient was 56 years old, the mean age reported in several papers on the beneficial effects of DBS, especially subthalamic nucleus (STN) stimulation in PD. Several studies found a less favorable outcome of bilateral STN stimulation in older compared to younger patients [1,2]. Most DBS studies have excluded patients above age 75. An age above 70 is considered as a relative contraindication and above 75 as an absolute contraindication. It is common sense that elderly patients will have more surgical complications (e.g. brain surgery in old age is more likely to be complicated by brain hemorrhage). Age is a cofactor for comorbidities as well as classical postoperative complications such as deep vein thrombosis or pulmonary infection. The cognitive reserve also changes with old age. Moreover, the non-dopaminergic motor signs such as dysarthria, dysphagia, postural instability, and gait disorders are also more prominent, thus decreasing the potential benefit as non-dopaminergic signs do not respond to surgery. Life expectancy is shorter in elderly patients, thereby also influencing the risk–benefit ratio.

Comorbidities

This patient's fair general health makes neurosurgery possible. Malignancies with markedly reduced life expectancy, unstable heart disease, active infection, marked subcortical arteriosclerotic encephalopathy, or other disabling cerebrovascular disease should be regarded as contraindications to DBS [3]. The borderline hypertension of this patient may increase the risk of intracranial bleeding. One study showed a more than 10-fold increase in cerebral hemorrhage in patients with preoperative vascular hypertension [4]. A thorough blood pressure investigation with possible antihypertensive treatment is needed before DBS.

Since the two most severe surgery-induced adverse effects are intracranial hematoma and infection, one should check for the absence of scalp infection and for use of any nonsteroidal anti-inflammatory drugs that promote bleeding, such as aspirin, anticoagulants, and lisuride.

Preoperative MRI screening is mandatory before any probe insertion in the brain to identify structural lesions with no clinical expression that could increase the risk of surgery. The mild changes seen in this patient's brain MRI were considered compatible with DBS although the risk of intracranial bleeding may be increased.

Neuropsychological and neuropsychiatric evaluation

Although DBS surgery has relatively few permanent cognitive side effects in well-selected young and non-demented patients [5], elderly patients or those with preoperative cognitive deterioration, risk permanent postoperative cognitive deterioration [6]. A thorough screening for cognitive deficits is thus mandatory. Neuropsychological evaluation with special emphasis on memory and executive function is highly recommended [7]. For evaluation of overall cognitive function, this patient was investigated with the Mattis Dementia Rating Scale (MDRS). His score was 131, which was considered low given his high educational level. A large test battery of executive function was applied, which confirmed a moderate frontal syndrome. As the MDRS score was similar 2 years previously, it was concluded that this impairment was stable and did not contraindicate surgery. In case of borderline scores, it is useful to repeat the evaluation after 1 year to verify that cognitive dysfunction has not progressed; progression could herald subcortical dementia which can be precipitated by surgery.

Mood changes and behavioral side effects are common after DBS surgery and occur especially in the first postoperative weeks or months [8]. Psychiatric symptoms that are disease-related must be distinguished from the psychiatric side effects of medication [9]. This patient had long interviews with a psychiatrist and a psychologist specialized in behavioral and affective symptoms that can occur in PD patients taking dopamine agonists. His mood and apathetic state were also studied with standardized scales and found normal. Only ongoing severe depression should be considered as absolute contraindication to surgery because of the risk of suicide [8]. It was concluded that this patient had developed a dopamine dysregulation syndrome while on high doses of pergolide, but that presently this syndrome had completely abated. Indeed, STN stimulation can be indicated in patients with hyperdopaminergic psychiatric symptoms thanks to the major decrease in dopaminergic drugs after STN stimulation [10]. Such patients are prone to develop perioperative psychiatric symptoms, however, and should be carefully followed during the postoperative year with adjustment of electrical parameters and drug doses according to both their motor and psychiatric states.

Motor evaluation

This patient fulfilled all the diagnostic criteria for PD, and 10-year duration ensures against an atypical form of parkinsonism. The best predictors of outcome from DBS are the magnitude of the motor response to levodopa and the quality of the "on" period [1,2,11]. Since this patient had minimal complaints related to parkinsonism at the peak effect of levodopa and was simultaneously disabled by dyskinesias and severe "off" periods, he can be considered an excellent candidate for surgery. A formal assessment using the Unified Parkinson's Disease Rating Scale (UPDRS) is mandatory, however, to evaluate worst-off/best-on motor function and the various types of dyskinesias, as recommended by the Core Assessment Program for Surgical Interventional Therapies in PD (CAPSIT-PD) protocol [12]. A suprathreshold dose of 250 mg of levodopa/carbidopa was given on an empty stomach in the morning after 12 h without dopaminergic treatment. The UPDRS motor score (from normal = 0 to maximal disability = 108) was 47 while "off" with severe akinetic-rigid right hemibody, and 7 while "on." Gait was severely impaired in "off" periods. The normalization of gait at the best levodopa effect with absence of freezing and imbalance was an indication for DBS. Dysarthria was, however, still present during "on" periods. The patient should be informed that DBS will not improve his speech, which may even deteriorate, whereas his "off" gait and dyskinesias have a good chance to improve greatly.

Socioeconomic status, expectations and cooperation

This divorced patient with no companion or children will be less well supported during the perioperative period and in the long term, which represents a negative factor for surgery, but not a contraindication. Moreover, surgery may not enable the patient to resume his professional activities, as this difficulty is related to his frontal lobe syndrome that will not be improved by DBS. A favorable point for DBS is, however, that this patient has no personality disorder and is cooperative. We should provide him a realistic explanation of what to expect from DBS, what the risks are, and we will check that these data match his expectations [13].

In conclusion, this patient fulfills the major criteria for DBS but will need intensive psychosocial support. The team neurosurgeon and anesthesiologist will be consulted finally to give the definitive agreement for neurosurgery.

Final diagnosis: PD with indication for DBS.

Pierre Pollak

References

1 Charles PD, Van Blercom N, Krack P *et al.* Predictors of effective bilateral subthalamic nucleus stimulation for PD. *Neurology* 2002; **59**: 932–4.

2 Welter ML, Houeto JL, Tezenas du Montcel S *et al.* Clinical predictive factors of subthalamic stimulation in Parkinson's disease. *Brain* 2002; **125**: 575–83.

3 Lang AE, Houeto JL, Krack P *et al.* Deep brain stimulation: Preoperative issues. *Mov Disord* 2006; **21**(S14): S171–96.

4 Gorgulho A, De Salles AA, Frighetto L, Behnke E. Incidence of hemorrhage associated with electrophysiological studies performed using macroelectrodes and microelectrodes in functional neurosurgery. *J Neurosurg* 2005; **102**: 888–96.

5 Ardouin C, Pillon B, Peiffer E *et al.* Bilateral subthalamic or pallidal stimulation for Parkinson's disease affects neither memory nor executive functions: a consecutive series of 62 patients. *Ann Neurol* 1999; **46**: 217–23.

6 Jarraya B, Bonnet AM, Duyckaerts C *et al.* Parkinson's disease, subthalamic stimulation, and selection of candidates: a pathological study. *Mov Disord* 2003; **18**: 1517–20.

7 Voon V, Kubu C, Krack P, Houeto JL, Troster AI. Deep brain stimulation: neuropsychological and neuropsychiatric issues. *Mov Disord* 2006; **21**(S14): S305–27.

8 Funkiewiez A, Ardouin C, Caputo E *et al.* Long-term effects of bilateral subthalamic nucleus stimulation on cognitive function, mood and behaviour in Parkinson's disease. *J Neurol Neurosurg Psychiatry* 2004; **75**: 834–9.

9 Lawrence AD, Evans AH, Lees AJ. Compulsive use of dopamine replacement therapy in Parkinson's disease: reward systems gone awry? *Lancet Neurol* 2003; **2**: 595–604.

10 Witjas T, Baunez C, Henry JM *et al.* Addiction in Parkinson's disease: impact of subthalamic nucleus deep brain stimulation. *Mov Disord* 2005; **20**: 1052–5.

11 Fraix V, Houeto JL, Lagrange C *et al.* Clinical and economic results of bilateral subthalamic nucleus stimulation in Parkinson's disease. *J Neurol Neurosurg Psychiatry* 2006; **77**: 443–9.

12 Defer GL, Widner H, Marie RM, Remy P, Levivier M. Core assessment program for surgical interventional therapies in Parkinson's disease (CAPSIT-PD). *Mov Disord* 1999; **14**: 572–84.

13 Schüpbach M, Gargiulo M, Welter ML *et al.* Neurosurgery in Parkinson disease: a distressed mind in a repaired body? *Neurology* 2006; **66**(12): 1811–16.

Case study 14

Case presentation

Mr L.C., a 71-year-old man whose Parkinson's disease (PD) had been evolving for 8 years, was referred to our clinic. The patient reported good initial response to antiparkinsonian therapy associating levodopa (150 mg × 3) and bromocriptine (15 mg × 3). But over the past few months, he had been suffering from a dysuria – treated with propanthelin (15 mg × 3) by his GP – forgetfulness, and difficulty in following several conversations. Despite his complaints, he was able to clearly describe his regular treatment: (1) Sinemet® 700 mg (Sinemet® 100 × 3 + Sinemet® LP 200 × 2); (2) Requip® 9 mg (3 × 1 mg, t.i.d.); (3) Comtan® 600 mg (200 mg × 3); and (4) Motilium® (30 mg).

The neurological examination showed amimia, dysarthria with hypophonia, and an akineto-hypertonic syndrome with a Unified Parkinson's Disease Rating Scale (UPDRS) score of 24 and a Hoehn & Yahr score of 2. The neuropsychological evaluation (see Table 3.14.1) showed:

• a decrease of global cognitive efficiency with a Mini Mental Status Examination (MMSE) score of 26 and a Mattis Dementia Rating Scale (MDRS) [1] score of 128/144

• a dysexecutive syndrome characterized by low lexical fluency (only five words beginning with S cited in one minute), a decreased ability to conceptualize (with only 3/6 categories achieved on the Wisconsin Card Sorting Test [WCST] and a low performance on the similarities test of the Frontal Assessment Battery [FAB] [2]) and a deficit of behavioral control (high number of abandons on WCST; low performance on the conflicting instructions section of the FAB)

• a retrieval deficit in episodic long-term memory as shown by a free- and cued-recall test [3] (with a low performance in free recall that was normalized by the semantic cues)

• visuoconstructive difficulties as shown by a spontaneous clock drawing test contrasting with a normal copy of the clock.

Table 3.14.1 Performance of patient L.C.

	L.C.	Abnormal values
Global efficiency		
Mini Mental Status Examination (/30)	26	< 26
Mattis Dementia Rating Scale (/144)	**128**	< 136
Executive functions		
Frontal Assessment Battery (/18)	**12**	< 16
Similarities (/3)	2	
Lexical fluency (/3)	1	
Motor series (/3)	2	
Conflicting instructions (/3)	2	
Go–no go (/3)	2	
Prehension behavior (/3)	3	
Wisconsin Card Sorting Test		
Criteria achieved (*n*) (/6)	**3**	< 6
Abandons (*n*)	**6**	
Perseverations (*n*)	3	
Memory		
Free- and Cued-Recall Test		
Free recall (/48)	**18**	< 27
Cued recall (/48)	46	< 44
Delayed free recall (/16)	**3**	<10
Delayed total recall (/16)	15	
Intrusions (*n*)	1	
Recognition (/16)	16	

Other cognitive functions assessed, including visuoperceptive, gestural, and linguistic functions, were not significantly impaired. Dysthymic features were noticed with the Montgomery–Asberg Depression Rating Scale.

Differential diagnosis

Cognitive changes are not infrequent in PD and the discussion should be based on the severity and the nature of the cognitive changes. In this patient, the changes are not severe enough to warrant a diagnosis of dementia, as shown by his MMSE and MDRS scores. Moreover, there was no impact on the patient's activities of daily living, such as the management of his own treatment. This ability to describe his treatment can be considered as an index of mental organization and functioning in a situation of daily living [4]. Therefore, these changes are consistent with the new concept of mild cognitive impairment in PD (PD-MCI) [5]. The proposal of isolating a subgroup of PD patients with mild cognitive changes can be useful for investigating the influence of specific factors such as higher age at onset or more severe parkinsonism on the cognitive performance of PD [6].

What might the lesions responsible for these cognitive changes in this patient be? From postmortem studies, it is now well established that neuronal PD lesions can be found outside the brain structures involved in motor control.

Such lesions are described either in subcortical (non-motor basal ganglia and mesencephalic nuclei) or cortical areas. (See review in [7] and [8].) The later lesions can be of the Alzheimer's type or consist in intracytoplasmic Lewy body inclusions. In our patient, the absence of a dementia syndrome and the late occurrence of cognitive impairment make it possible to rule out the diagnosis of dementia with Lewy bodies. In the same way, the nature of the cognitive changes reported in this observation makes it very unlikely that the patient has a superimposed Alzheimer's disease (AD), even at an early predementia stage. Indeed, the retrieval deficit described here is characteristic of a fronto-striatal dysfunction and differs from the hippocampal amnestic disorders of AD where semantic cues only marginally improve the free-recall deficit [9].

In fact, the cognitive changes observed in this patient are typical of those seen in PD characterized by a marked dysexecutive syndrome with a retrieval deficit. They mainly result from the subcortical lesions of the disease involving the basal ganglia and/or the long ascending cholinergic and monoaminergic subcortico-cortical systems. The dysfunction induced by the brain lesions may also be aggravated here by the presence of: (1) medication with anticholinergic properties, such as propanthelin which can cross the blood–brain barrier and specifically interact with attention and executive functions in PD patients [10], and (2) depression which also impacts on performance in executive functions as shown by Starkstein *et al.* [11].

Final diagnosis: mild cognitive impairment in PD.

Discussion

PD-MCI is frequently observed and is mainly characterized by a dysexecutive syndrome responsible for forgetfulness owing to a difficulty to activate retrieval strategies. These executive functions refer to the processes that are needed for the completion of complex cognitive tasks requiring, for example, to select the information to be processed, to find the rule to apply, to shift mental sets, to resist cognitive interferences, or to actively self-retrieve information from memory. Most of these processes are strongly correlated with *working memory*, defined as the ability to maintain and manipulate pertinent information during a brief period of time and to use this internal representation to elaborate a program of response. Miyake *et al.* [12] highlighted that among the executive processes, the unitary ones are: (1) mental set shifting, (2) information updating and monitoring, and (3) inhibition of reflexive responses. The executive functions can be assessed by distinctive questionnaires or tests (see Table 3.14.2).

Given the close interconnections between the basal ganglia and prefrontal cortical areas, it is not surprising that neurodegenerative disorders that primarily involve these subcortical structures can induce frontal-related syndrome, and particularly an executive dysfunction. When present, it is important to check the absence of any confounding factors such as anticholinergic therapy or depression. It is important to bear in mind that PD-MCI may evolve

Table 3.14.2 Executive functions and their assessment

Executive functions	Neuropsychological assessment
Volition	
Motivation	Apathy Scale
Initiation	Neuropsychiatric Inventory
Planning	
Working memory	Digit Ordering Test
Conceptualization	Wisconsin Card Sorting Test
Execution	Verbal fluency
Set activation	Free- and Cued-Recall Test
Flexibility	Trail Making Test
Maintenance	Stroop Test
Control	
Awareness and insight	Questionnaires
Cognitive evaluation	Reward Associative Learning
Behavioral autonomy	Prehension, behavior

toward full-blown dementia, especially when the patient is over 70 years old and has a long disease duration. Additional risk factors are more severe parkinsonism (in particular rigidity, postural instability, and gait disturbances), low lexical fluency, and a diminished response to levodopa therapy, all signs that indicate a diffusion of brain lesions. Therefore, Mr L.C. is highly at risk of developing dementia in the near future.

Bruno Dubois, Virginie Czernecki

References

1 Mattis S. *Dementia Rating Scale. Professional manual.* Odessa, FL: Psychological Assessment Resources Inc, 1988.
2 Dubois B, Slachevsky A, Litvan I, Pillon B. The FAB: a Frontal Assessment Battery at bedside. *Neurology* 2000; **55**(11): 1621–6.
3 Grober E, Buschke H. Genuine memory deficits in dementia. *Dev Neuropsychol* 1987; **3**: 13–36.
4 Dubois B, Burn D, Goetz C et al. Diagnostic procedures for Parkinson's disease dementia: recommendations from the Movement Disorder Society task force. *Mov Disord* 2007; **22**(16): 2314–24.
5 Caviness JN, Driver-Dunckley E, Connor DJ et al. Defining mild cognitive impairment in Parkinson's disease. *Mov Disord* 2007; **22**(9): 1272–7.
6 Dubois B. Is PD-MCI a useful concept? *Mov Disord* 2007; **22**(9): 1215–16.
7 Pillon B, Boller F, Levy R, Dubois B. Cognitive deficits and dementia in Parkinson's disease. In: F Boller, J Grafman (eds). *Handbook of Neuropsychology*, Vol. 6. *Aging and dementia.* Amsterdam: Elsevier, 2001; 311–71.
8 Emre M. What causes mental dysfunction in Parkinson's disease? *Mov Disord* 2003; **18**(Suppl 6): S63–71.
9 Pillon B, Deweer B, Agid Y, Dubois B. Explicit memory in Alzheimer's, Huntington's, and Parkinson's diseases. *Arch Neurol* 1993; **50**(4): 374–9.

10 Dubois B, Pillon B, Lhermitte F, Agid Y. Cholinergic deficiency and frontal dysfunction in Parkinson's disease. *Ann Neurol* 1990; **28**(2): 117–21.

11 Starkstein SE, Preziosi TJ, Berthier ML, Bolduc PL, Mayberg HS, Robinson RG. Depression and cognitive impairment in Parkinson's disease. *Brain* 1989; **112**(Pt 5): 1141–53.

12 Miyake A, Friedman NP, Emerson MJ, Witzki AH, Howerter A, Wager TD. The unity and diversity of executive functions and their contributions to complex 'frontal lobe' tasks: a latent variable analysis. *Cognit Psychol* 2000; **41**(1): 49–100.

Case presentation

A 60-year-old right-handed man was referred for evaluation at a movement disorders center after being diagnosed with Parkinson's disease (PD) during a hospitalization 1 month earlier. The patient's family reported that he had been in his usual state of health until approximately 6 months earlier. At that time he was living alone and taking care of himself. His family reported that since then, however, he had progressively deteriorated mentally and physically.

Four months ago, the patient was brought to his local emergency room with a complaint of palpitations. He was admitted for evaluation. He denied depression but on examination his affect appeared flat. Heart rate was 80 beats per minute with a regular rate and rhythm and no murmurs, rubs, or gallops. Chest X-ray, blood work, and electrocardiogram were normal. He was diagnosed as having an anxiety attack and was treated with alprazolam 0.25 mg/ day. He was also started on sertraline and titrated up to 150 mg/day for possible depression.

Over the next few months he experienced increasing confusion and short-term memory difficulty. The family reported that when he went to renew his driver's license, he became confused and thought that he was being asked about illicit drugs rather than his prescription medications. His license was not renewed. His family found this episode surprising and out of character. In addition, his family reported that he saw people and heard voices at home at night a few times a week. He grew increasingly apathetic and his daily food intake declined.

The patient was hospitalized again 1 month ago for weight loss and decreased appetite. He also reported fatigue, memory difficulty, and a few falls. Computed tomography scan of the brain was normal and magnetic resonance imaging (MRI) revealed mild microvascular ischemic changes involving the deep white matter of the cerebrum. He was examined by a neurologist who noted moderately slow movements, masked face, mild postural reflex impairment, and executive function difficulty. A diagnosis of PD was made and he was started on carbidopa/levodopa 25/100 t.i.d. with mild improvement in movement. He was no longer able to live independently, however, and moved in with his daughter.

At his initial evaluation with the movement disorder specialist, his family reported that his movements were mildly improved with carbidopa/levodopa and his depression and anxiety were fairly well controlled on sertraline 150 mg/day. His daughter reported that his cognitive abilities varied through the day and at times he stared off into space. Past medical history included diabetes, hyperlipidemia, hypotension, insomnia, and sexual dysfunction. On review of systems, he reported mild swallowing difficulties associated with occasional coughing. He also reported ongoing insomnia and constipation. His Mini Mental State Examination score was 26. He could name the president and vice president, but could only recall one of three objects at five minutes. He had difficulty with abstract concepts and comprehending new information.

On neurological examination, he was seen to have mildly decreased facial expression, moderate hypophonia, and mild micrographia. Extraocular movements were normal. Fine coordinated movements of the hands and fingers were moderately decreased on the right and moderate-to-markedly reduced on the left. Tone was slightly increased in both upper extremities, moderately increased in both lower extremities, and normal in the neck. Stride length was mildly shortened, posture was slightly flexed, and balance was normal. Arm swing during ambulation was absent on the left and moderately decreased on the right.

Differential diagnosis

The differential diagnosis for this case includes dementia with Lewy bodies (DLB), Parkinson's disease with dementia (PDD), Alzheimer disease (AD), vascular dementia, progressive supranuclear palsy (PSP), multiple system atrophy (MSA), and frontotemporal dementia (FTD). The key features of the case that make DLB the most likely diagnosis include the concurrent development of progressive dementia and parkinsonism, visual hallucinations, and fluctuating cognition.

DLB is the second most common form of dementia after AD. The diagnosis can be challenging owing to the potential clinical overlap with other dementias, and definitive diagnosis is dependent on autopsy confirmation. McKeith *et al.* revised the criteria for DLB in 2005 and included a central feature, core features, suggestive features, and supportive features. The central feature required for the diagnosis is dementia with progressive cognitive decline. Deficits on tests of attention, executive dysfunction, and visuospatial ability may be prominent. Core features include spontaneous parkinsonism, recurrent visual hallucinations, and fluctuating cognition with variations in attention and alertness. Suggestive features include positron emission tomography or single photon emission computed tomography imaging demonstrating loss of dopamine neurons in the striatum, rapid eye movement (REM) sleep behavior disorder (RBD), and severe neuroleptic sensitivity. Two or more core features or one core feature plus at least one suggestive feature are diagnostic of probable DLB. In addition, in DLB dementia precedes or is concurrent with parkinsonism, whereas in PDD dementia emerges in the context of well-established PD. Typically, in DLB the dementia should begin no more than 1 year after the onset of parkinsonism.

Formal criteria for PDD have not been established. Dementia and hallucinations are late features of PD, usually occurring several years after the onset of motor signs, although subtle cognitive impairment is not uncommon in early PD. The risk of dementia in PD increases with increasing age and duration of parkinsonism. PDD and DLB are both associated with α-synuclein pathology in the limbic and neocortical brain areas and share a high incidence of visual hallucinations and RBD. In addition, the overall pattern of cognitive impairment and fluctuations in attention are similar. Whether PDD and DLB represent the same or different disease processes has not yet been defined and the cutoff for onset of dementia within 1 year of motor signs in DLB is arbitrary.

AD is by far the most common cause of dementia. A diagnosis of probable AD requires deficits in two or more areas of cognition, including memory, that progressively worsen and are not caused by delirium or other systemic or brain illnesses. To a large extent, AD remains a diagnosis of exclusion. Older series reported parkinsonism in as many as 30% of AD patients, but with improvements in staining techniques for Lewy bodies it is now thought that most if not all of these patients actually have DLB. Hallucinations occur in up 50% of AD patients and delusions in up to 75%, but are generally later features of the disease. In the case described, parkinsonism and hallucinations were early features.

Vascular dementia occurs when cerebrovascular disease results in brain injury that disrupts networks for memory and thinking. It is a heterogeneous disorder that can be related to a variety of vascular risk factors and caused by various types of vascular injury. The profile of cognitive impairment varies based on the pattern of brain injury. There are many proposed criteria that vary in their sensitivity and specificity. All require evidence of dementia, vascular brain injury, and a presumed causal relationship between the vascular brain injury and the dementia. Helpful diagnostic features may include abrupt onset, stepwise progression, history of stroke, focal neurological signs, and perhaps most importantly, evidence of cerebrovascular disease that can reasonably be judged to be etiologically related to the dementia. In the case described, there was no history of stroke, there appeared to be progressive rather than stepwise worsening, and the ischemic disease identified on MRI was unlikely to explain the parkinsonism or dementia. Furthermore, unprovoked visual hallucinations are rare in vascular dementia.

PSP and MSA are atypical parkinsonisms characterized by relatively symmetric parkinsonism with little or no response to levodopa, and early speech and balance difficulty. Clinical criteria for possible PSP include vertical supranuclear gaze palsy or both slowing of vertical saccades and prominent postural instability with falls within the first year. Early onset of cognitive impairment is a supportive feature of PSP. MSA is associated with a combination of parkinsonism, autonomic, cerebellar, and corticospinal dysfunction. Functionally important cognitive impairment is not considered part of MSA. Hallucinations unrelated to medication rule out both PSP and MSA. The patient described did not exhibit abnormalities of eye movement, prominent postural instability, cerebellar, or corticospinal dysfunction, and did experience visual hallucinations unrelated to medication.

FTD is characterized by prominent behavioral changes that herald the onset of dementia. These may include social disinhibition, apathy, overeating, repetitive motor behaviors, and loss of judgment and insight. Early cognitive dysfunction includes deficits in executive and language ability with relatively preserved memory. Parkinsonian features may occur later in the disease. Frontotemporal dementia and parkinsonism linked to chromosome 17 (FTDP-17) is a rare autosomal dominant neurodegenerative disorder. It presents as an atypical parkinsonism and is frequently associated with falls and supranuclear gaze palsy. Additional characteristic features include positive family history, progressive neuropsychiatric disturbances, and poorly controlled seizure disorder.

In the case described, the patient experienced concurrent dementia and parkinsonism with progressive decline. He also experienced visual (and auditory) hallucinations early in the course of the illness that were not induced by medications. The history revealed fluctuations in cognition with episodes of confusion and decreased attention. He did not exhibit eye movement abnormalities, prominent postural instability with falls, or cerebellar or corticospinal signs. Ischemic lesions on MRI did not appear to account for his parkinsonism or dementia. He was therefore diagnosed with probable DLB.

Final diagnosis: dementia with Lewy bodies.

Discussion

Treatment of DLB is symptomatic. To date, there is no proven treatment to slow or modify the disease. This patient was treated with alprazolam and sertraline with good control of anxiety and depression. Quetiapine 25 mg q.h.s. was added and hallucinations resolved. In DLB, the response of parkinsonian motor features to levodopa is quite variable and patients are less likely to exhibit a robust and sustained response compared to patients with PD. This patient had a modest improvement in parkinsonism with carbidopa/levodopa 25/100 t.i.d., and the dose was slowly escalated to 25/100 two tablets q.i.d. with modest additional motor benefit. Acetylcholinesterase inhibitors have not been well studied for the treatment of dementia in DLB, but a severe cholinergic deficit is often present. Therefore, the decision was made to start the patient on rivastigmine transdermal patch and his response will be monitored clinically.

Terry McClain, Robert A. Hauser

Further reading

Aarsland D, Brønnick K, Ehrt U *et al*. Neuropsychiatric symptoms in patients with Parkinson's disease and dementia: frequency, profile and associated care giver stress. *J Neurol Neurosurg Psychiatry* 2007; **78**: 36–42.

Boeve BF. Parkinson-related dementias. *Neurol Clin* 2007; 25(3): 761–81.

Chui H, Nielsen-Brown N. Vascular cognitive impairment. Continuum: lifelong learning in neurology. *Dementia* 2007; **13**(2): 109–43.

Dubois B, Feldman HH, Jacova C *et al*. Research criteria for the diagnosis of Alzheimer's disease: revising the NINCDS-ADRDA criteria. *Lancet Neurol* 2007; **6**(8): 734–46.

Farlow MR. Alzheimer's disease. Continuum: lifelong learning in neurology. *Dementia* 2007; **13**(2): 39–68.

Galasko DR. Dementia with Lewy bodies. Continuum: lifelong learning in neurology. *Dementia* 2007; **13**(2): 69–86.

Graff-Radford N. Normal pressure hydrocephalus. Continuum: lifelong learning in neurology. *Dementia* 2007; **13**(2): 144–64.

Lippa CF, Duda JE, Grossman M *et al*. DLB and PDD boundary issues: diagnosis, treatment, molecular pathology, and biomarkers. *Neurology* 2007; **68**: 812–19.

McKeith IG, Dickson DW, Lowe J *et al*. Diagnosis and management of dementia with Lewy bodies. Third report of the DLB consortium. *Neurology* 2005; **65**: 1863–72.

Monza D, Ciano C, Scaioli V *et al*. Neurophysiological features in relation to clinical signs in clinically diagnosed corticobasal degeneration. *Neurol Sci* 2003; **24**(1): 16–23.

Sha S, Hou C, Viskontas IV, Miller BL. Are frontotemporal lobar degeneration, progressive supranuclear palsy and corticobasal degeneration distinct diseases? *Nat Clin Pract Neurol* 2006; **2**(12): 658–65.

Viskontas I, Miller B. Frontotemporal dementia. Continuum: lifelong learning in neurology. *Dementia* 2007; **13**(2): 87–108.

Wenning G, Geser F. Diagnosis and treatment of multiple system atrophy: an update. *Adv Clin Neurosci Rehabil* 2004; **3**(6): 5–10.

Zesiewicz TA, Baker MJ, Dunne PB, Hauser RA. Diffuse Lewy body disease. *Curr Treat Options Neurol* 2001; **3**(6): 507–18.

Case study 16

Case presentation

This 60-year-old man had developed a tremor of his right arm at the age of 53, spreading 2 years later to his left arm and legs. He also developed mild side-to-side head tremor. After another 2 years, he started to slow down and noticed that his writing was becoming slow and tremulous and his voice strained. His walking was slow and he easily fatigued. His father and two of five siblings had previously been diagnosed with Parkinson's disease (PD), all having a tremor disorder with onset at age 40–60.

On examination at age 59, he had facial hypomimia and adductor dysphonia. He had an asymmetrical tremor present at rest involving all four limbs, more marked in the right arm with intermittent pill-rolling of the right hand. Tremor was also present on posture and became more pronounced on action, particularly when writing and drawing a spiral. Increase of tone was moderate in his legs, and mild in his arms. He had slowness and irregularity of alternating movements, but no clear fatiguing or decrement. On walking, he had diminished arm swing which was more pronounced on the left side. A levodopa challenge with up to 1000 mg over a period of 4 weeks did not improve tremor. Additional investigations including brain magnetic resonance imaging (MRI) and DaTSCAN™ were all normal.

Differential diagnosis

With onset of tremor at this age, the first diagnoses to consider would be PD, essential tremor (ET) and dystonic tremor (DT). With regard to PD, the cardinal feature apart from rigidity and tremor is of course bradykinesia. Pointers towards PD in this patient are the onset of a rest tremor in one arm spreading within 2 years to the other side and also involving the legs, as well as the general slowing of movements including gait, handwriting, and reduced arm swing. Postural tremor also occurs in PD and typically this is a faster re-emergent tremor at 6–8 Hz compared to the pill-rolling rest tremor at 3–5 Hz.

ET is characterized by a fairly symmetrical postural tremor of the arms, often associated with a positive family history and with a good response of the tremor to alcohol. ET has a bimodal distribution with onset peaks in the second and sixth decades [1,2]. Overall prevalence ranges from 305 to 1700/100 000. Patients with onset > 60 years have a faster progression than those with young onset. The subgroup with marked head/voice tremor has a positive association with female sex. According to the accepted definition, "essential" tremor should have no associated features [3]. Hence true parkinsonism or dystonia should not be seen in typical ET. Some authors, however, describe an association with dystonia (cervical dystonia, spasmodic dysphonia, or writer's cramp) in up to 47% of their patients with ET [2], whereas others exclude patients with concomitant dystonia [1].

Another debate is whether patients with ET are at increased risk of PD. This link is supported by the observation that in some PD patients, a long-standing postural tremor precedes the onset of parkinsonism by years or even decades and that dopamine transporter imaging was abnormal in some patients diagnosed with ET. Olfaction has also been reported to be reduced in ET compared to controls. Because different diagnostic criteria have been applied, ET is probably a heterogeneous disorder with differences in sex distribution, rate of progression and anatomic distribution of tremor, as well as the associated features. This heterogeneity is probably the reason why linkage has been found to three different loci [4] with a susceptibility variant (Ser9Gly) in the dopamine D$_3$ receptor gene (*DRD3*), but no gene has as yet been found.

It has been speculated that ET is overdiagnosed and that some subgroups have another condition. In our patient, pointers towards ET would be a tremor with a postural component, neck and voice involvement, and a positive family history. Pointers against ET are the marked asymmetry of tremor and the presence of rest tremor from onset. Although rest tremor has been described in ET, the occurrence is associated with more severe and advanced stages [5]. General slowing with reduced arm swing is also atypical for ET.

The examination of this patient revealed some pointers or "red flags" against the diagnosis of PD. Finger tapping was slow, but the patient did not have true bradykinesia as defined in the UK Parkinson's Disease Society Brain Bank (PDSBB) diagnostic criteria, which states that apart from slowness of initiation of voluntary movement, there should be a "progressive reduction in speed and amplitude of repetitive actions." It is worth pointing out that testing bradykinesia in a patient by finger tapping can be difficult as tremor can supervene and be mistaken as decrement. Tremor of head and voice as well as the immediate worsening of the tremor on action is uncommon in PD although head tremor has been described. The immediate worsening of the tremor on postures or action as well as worsening when writing and drawing a spiral points away from typical PD tremor and rather suggests a dystonic component. Finally the lack of response to an adequate dose of levodopa (1000 mg for 4 weeks) raises doubts about the diagnosis of PD.

The constellation of prominent tremor with only mild non-tremor components of parkinsonism and absence of gait disorder with a slower disease progression and a tremor which is refractory to medications including maximally tolerated levodopa has also been called "benign tremulous parkinsonism" [6,7]. Although disease progression is very slow, the term benign is misleading because in most cases tremor has a prominent action component that impairs eating and writing and can, therefore, cause marked disability. There is much uncertainty as to whether this diagnosis only represents one end of the bell-shaped curve of typical PD or if it may represent a unique disorder.

A third possibility in this patient is dystonic tremor (DT). Symptoms and signs in favor of this diagnosis are asymmetric or unilateral tremor with a resting component early on, neck and voice involvement, and the characteristic position- or task-specificity (writing or drawing a spiral). This entity is under-recognized and often misdiagnosed as PD or ET. It should be recognized that patients with DT often have a rest tremor, sometimes even with classical pill-rolling, jaw tremor, facial hypomimia, and impaired arm swing in the affected arm – all features that may suggest PD to the unwary [8]. In addition, some dystonia patients have increased limb tone (distinct from cogwheeling alone in a tremulous limb). This does not necessarily equate with parkinsonian rigidity, but it may be difficult to make a distinction. What such patients do not have is true akinesia, as defined by progressive fatiguing and decrement of alternating repetitive movements. Dystonia may be present in patients in parkinsonism, and may sometimes be a presenting feature, but this applies mostly to patients with early-onset PD.

In comparison to ET, patients with DT tend to have more asymmetric or unilateral, involvement, more position- and task-specificity, more frequent neck involvement, and additional presence of dystonia. They also seem to display intermittent "flurries" of tremor more often. Following the Movement Disorder Society consensus criteria, our patient matched the diagnosis of "tremor associated with dystonia (laryngeal dystonia was present)" [3]. Presynaptic dopaminergic deficit (and hence PD) was ruled out with a normal DaTSCAN™.

Emphasizing this clinical diagnostic difficulty are the results in two *de novo* clinical trials in patients with a clinical diagnosis of early PD, where 11–15% of patients studied had normal nigrostriatal uptake of presynaptic ligands. Thus, in the REAL-PET study, 21 (11%) of the patients enrolled in the imaging substudy had normal fluorodopa positron emission tomography (PET) scans, and in the 19 in whom the scans were repeated 2 years later, they were again normal [9]. In the ELLDOPA study, 21 (14.7%) patients scanned with ^{123}I-FP-CIT had scans without evidence of dopaminergic deficit (SWEDDs), and follow-up scans remained normal in patients rescanned after 4 years [10]. In the ELLDOPA trial, patients with SWEDDs did not respond to levodopa. Since DaTSCAN™ is the gold standard to reveal presynaptic dopaminergic deficit with high sensitivity, this relatively high percentage of patients with SWEDDs suggests a diagnosis other than PD. These patients may have ET or more likely dystonic tremor as many have subtle features of dystonia which can be missed [8].

Final diagnosis: dystonic tremor.

Treatment

Treatment of DT is challenging and difficult. Levodopa is generally ineffective. Drugs used for ET (propranolol, primidone) could be tried, but in our experience are generally unhelpful. Anticholinergics may produce side effects which outweigh the benefits, especially given that most patients with SWEDDs are in their sixties or seventies. Deep brain stimulation may turn out to be the most valuable option in such patients, but the best target (thalamus, pallidum, or indeed subthalamic nucleus) has yet to be defined.

Georg H. Kägi, Kailash P. Bhatia

References

1 Bain PG, Findley LJ, Thompson PD *et al.* A study of hereditary essential tremor. *Brain* 1994; **117**: 805–24.
2 Lou JS, Jankovic J. Essential tremor: clinical correlates in 350 patients. *Neurology* 1991; **41**: 234–8.
3 Deuschl G, Bain P, Brin M. Consensus statement of the Movement Disorder Society on Tremor. Ad Hoc Scientific Committee. *Mov Disord* 1998; **13**(Suppl 3): 2–23.
4 Deng H, Le W, Jankovic J. Genetics of essential tremor. *Brain* 2007; **130**: 1456–64.
5 Cohen O, Pullman S, Jurewicz E, Watner D, Louis ED. Rest tremor in patients with essential tremor: prevalence, clinical correlates, and electrophysiologic characteristics. *Arch Neurol* 2003; **60**: 405–10.
6 Josephs KA, Matsumoto JY, Ahlskog JE. Benign tremulous parkinsonism. *Arch Neurol* 2006; **63**: 354–7.
7 Marshall V, Grosset DG. Role of dopamine transporter imaging in the diagnosis of atypical tremor disorders. *Mov Disord* 2003; **18**(Suppl 7): S22–7.
8 Schneider SA, Edwards MJ, Mir P *et al.* Patients with adult-onset dystonic tremor resembling parkinsonian tremor have scans without evidence of dopaminergic deficit (SWEDDs). *Mov Disord* 2007; **22**(15): 2210–15.
9 Whone AL, Watts RL, Stoessl AJ *et al.*; REAL-PET Study Group. Slower progression of Parkinson's disease with ropinirole versus levodopa: the REAL-PET study. *Ann Neurol* 2003; **54**: 93–101.
10 Fahn S, Oakes D, Shoulson I *et al.*; Parkinson Study Group. Levodopa and the progression of Parkinson's disease. *N Engl J Med* 2004; **351**: 2498–508.

Case study 17

Case presentation

A 78-year-old man was referred to our Movement Disorders Unit by his family physician because of gait difficulties. The patient's main complaint was fatigue after walking 100 m. He experienced no leg pain or sensory abnormalities while walking and denied any chest pain or dyspnea. He also reported having become slow in all activities and especially in walking. Neurological examination revealed a positive palmomental reflex with no other primitive reflexes, left central facial palsy, and positive Babinski sign on the left. Speech was slow and monotonous but intelligible, with no dysarthria or dysphonia. Other findings included psychomotor slowing, hypomimia, and mild rigidity of the hands, with no tremor. Limb movements were slow, as was his gait. The patient had to use the arm rest of the chair to stand up. While walking, he took short steps with mild stooped posture and postural instability. There was no associated hand tilt. Freezing of gait was not noted. The patient's score on the Mini Mental State Examination (MMSE) was 27/30.

Brain magnetic resonance imaging demonstrated diffuse white-matter periventricular hypodensities, and multiple bilateral infarcts in the cortex and subcortex. The ventricles were mildly dilated, and there was also mild cortical atrophy.

Differential diagnosis

The patient had definite parkinsonian symptoms combined with pyramidal signs and positive primitive developmental reflexes. The differential diagnosis of parkinsonism is broad, but in this case it could be narrowed down fairly quickly. Some of the most common causes of parkinsonism in the elderly, namely medications, normal pressure hydrocephalus (NPH), diffuse Lewy body disease, and progressive supranuclear palsy, were easily ruled out. The patient did not use any of the drugs known to induce parkinsonism (e.g. dopamine receptor blocking agents, valproic acid, selective serotonin reuptake inhibitors, or calcium channel antagonists). The clinical examination and brain imaging findings were not compatible with NPH. Also, the features typical to parkinsonian syndromes (gaze palsy, hallucinations, dementia, recurrent falls) were absent. Multisystem atrophy (MSA) was also unlikely, despite the symmetry of symptoms and the presence of pyramidal signs, as the patient did not present with recurrent falls, and the autonomic and/or cerebellar signs required for the diagnosis of MSA were absent. Therefore, the remaining diagnostic possibilities were Parkinson's disease (PD) or vascular parkinsonism (VP).

PD generally appears in the fifth or sixth decade, but onset in the elderly is not rare. By contrast, the incidence of VP increases with age. In general, VP accounts for an estimated 3–6% of all cases of parkinsonism [1]. Clinico-ana-tomical studies of patients with a presumed diagnosis of PD revealed patho-logical criteria for VP in 11% [2]. The two entities may also coexist in the same patient. Their clinical differentiation is based on the presence of risk factors, symptoms and signs on examination, and neuroimaging.

Risk factors

Several studies have shown that VP is characterized by a male preponderance, older age at onset, and high frequency of vascular risk factors, especially hy-pertension and diabetes mellitus, followed by hyperlipidemia, ischemic heart disease, and documented cerebral stroke. Vascular risk factors have been found to be prevalent in elderly patients with mild parkinsonian signs, espe-cially rigidity. They were noted in 83% of patients with VP compared to only 31% of patients with PD [3]. Moreover, vascular risk factors occur significantly less often in patients with idiopathic PD than in age-matched controls.

Clinical phenotype

Fatigue is one of the most frequent complaints of patients with PD and other forms of parkinsonism. It should be emphasized, however, that fatigue in gen-eral is a non-specific symptom, and fatigue while walking is very common in systemic diseases, especially congestive heart failure. In patients with heart failure, however, fatigue is usually accompanied by chest pain and is relieved by rest. Early fatigue while walking is also characteristic of lumbar spinal ste-nosis, but in these cases it is usually associated with back and thigh pain that is also rapidly alleviated by rest.

The presence of pyramidal signs in our patient was the first indication of the diagnosis of VP. Pyramidal signs, usually a positive Babinski sign and hyper-reflexia on the more affected side, can also be present in PD, and bilateral posi-tive plantar reflexes may also be present in MSA, but in the absence of facial palsy, spastic dysarthria, and limb weakness. Additional signs of VP, though not fully present in our patient, are positive frontal release signs, cognitive deterioration, personality changes, and pseudobulbar signs. Acute onset and step-like progression of the disease course are considered a hallmark of VP, but are actually reported in only 25% of cases [4]. A history of step-like progression of signs and symptoms has been documented in only five pathologically proven cases of VP [5]. On the basis of a large clinical study, Winikates & Jankovic [4] proposed that the clinical phenotype of VP is heterogenous and includes one form with acute onset (possibly associated with basal ganglia infarctions) and another with insidious progression (possibly associated with a more diffuse subcortical white matter ischemia). This assumption was partially confirmed by the clinicopathological study of Zijlmans *et al.* [6] in patients with a pathological diagnosis of VP where macroscopic lacunae in the basal ganglia or thalamus were observed in 4/4 patients with a progressive onset of parkinsonism after an acute hemiparetic stroke. These findings were also noted, however, in nearly half the patients (7/13) with an insidious onset of parkinsonism.

It is generally accepted that the main feature of VP is bilateral symmetric parkinsonism affecting mainly the lower limbs; hence, the synonym "lower body parkinsonism." By contrast, PD is generally characterized by tremor and/or rigidity and/or bradykinesia that starts in one hand, progresses to the unilateral leg, and then to the contralateral side. Furthermore, the involved limbs in VP show bradykinesia and rigidity but not tremor, either resting or postural. Nevertheless, several studies have reported an atypical tremor and even rest tremor in up to 20% of patients who were diagnosed with VP according to clinical and radiological criteria [3,5,7]. Indeed, in one study, postural tremor was more common in patients with VP than in patients with PD [3]. Therefore, the diagnosis of VP cannot be excluded by the presence of tremor.

The limb rigidity in VP is sometimes difficult to define as it might be a combination of lead-pipe rigidity, spasticity, or paratonia owing to the involvement of the frontal lobe and pyramidal tract. Since the incidence of rigidity and bradykinesia is similar in VP and PD, their presence does not aid in the differentiation of these entities.

The gait disorder in VP dominates the clinical phenotype. The clinical description varies from a classic slow, shuffling gait with short steps, to a broad-based gait with postural instability, start hesitation, and freezing. Stooped posture might be present, but is generally mild and does not reach the magnitude seen in patients with PD and camptocormia. Postural instability and falls are common as presenting symptoms in VP, whereas they tend to appear at a later stage in patients with PD [3].

Imaging studies
A finding of vascular lesions on brain imaging is mandatory for the diagnosis of VP; however, it does not always exclude other coexisting pathologies. Ischemic brain lesions have also been observed in patients with clinico-anatomically proven PD; some studies even reported higher rates than in controls [3,8]. It is important to grade the vascular lesions and define their location to establish a cause-and-effect relationship. Solitary cortical or subcortical infarcts do not cause the same symptomatology as widespread small-vessel disease. Critchley [9] was the first to propose that multiple vascular lesions

in the basal ganglia are responsible for what he termed "arteriosclerotic parkinsonism." Since then, efforts have been made to link the location and extent of the vascular lesions to the clinical phenotype. The vascular lesions in VP are located in the cortical and subcortical gray matter (especially the basal ganglia), in the subcortical white matter, or diffusely in the frontal and periventricular white matter. Widespread lesions in the frontal white matter seem to be more closely related to VP than lesions in the basal ganglia [7]. Furthermore, involvement of more than one vascular territory is common in VP [4,10]. Frontal atrophy and white matter lucencies are also a common finding, but may be less specific.

Taken together, in this patient, the presence of vascular risk factors, the clinical phenotype of symmetrical onset of bradykinesia and rigidity, the lack of tremor, the presence of unilateral pyramidal signs, and the positive imaging findings make VP the most likely diagnosis.

Final diagnosis: vascular parkinsonism.

Diagnosis confirmation

Nuclear imaging

^{123}I-FP-CIT single photon emission computed tomography (SPECT) can be used to distinguish presynaptic from postsynaptic dopaminergic impairment. The ligand ^{123}I-FP-CIT binds with high affinity to the presynaptic dopamine transporters. Therefore, since VP is theoretically a pathologically postsynaptic dopaminergic disorder, findings on nuclear imaging with a presynaptic marker should be normal. By contrast, in PD, which is basically a presynaptic dopaminergic disorder and has a predominantly asymmetric onset, a corresponding asymmetric reduction in ligand uptake is to be expected. These assumptions were supported by studies of patients who fulfilled the clinical criteria for VP, in whom normal or near-normal presynaptic tracer binding was noted on SPECT imaging [11]. Other studies, however, reported a significant presynaptic dopaminergic deficit in patients with VP who had an insidious or acute onset of parkinsonism, affecting the striatum in the same manner as described in PD, though more symmetrically [12].

The inconsistency among these studies has several possible explanations. First, as VP and PD are both common entities, multi-infarcts may coexist in the same patient, with the Lewy body pathology being the cause of the reduced ligand uptake. Alternatively, strategic infarcts in the substantia nigra and/or striatum may disrupt the basal ganglia motor output or the thalamocortical pathways and cause a presynaptic decrease in ligand uptake. Therefore, a different pattern of the vascular ischemic changes among the studies might explain the opposing results of studies with clinicoradiological correlation. Faulty diagnosis and the effect of medications on ligand uptake might also play a role. Postsynaptic D2 receptor SPECT or positron emission tomography (PET) imaging might be useful for complete visualization of the dopaminergic system within the striatum, but thus far only a few studies have evaluated the role of this technique in VP, and the conclusions were equivocal. Interestingly, a study evaluating the clinical features of patients with a clinical diagnosis of VP against the imaging findings yielded no clinical differences between patients with normal and abnormal scans [13]. Another nuclear imaging technique that might be useful for distinguishing PD from VP is cardiac ^{123}I-meta-iodobenzylguanidine (MIBG) scintigraphy. One study reported myocardial postganglionic sympathetic dysfunction in patients with PD, but not in most patients with VP.

Other measures

Patients with PD and other neurodegenerative parkinsonian syndromes have markedly impaired olfactory functions, even in the very early stages of the disease. This corresponds to the neuropathological findings of Lewy bodies in the anterior olfactory nucleus. Olfactory function is substantially better in VP, and no different from that in elderly healthy patients. Therefore, tests for sense of smell might serve as an adjunctive diagnostic tool.

Treatment

The management of patients with VP is based on secondary prevention and symptomatic treatment. Hypertension, diabetes, and hyperlipidemia must be controlled and treatment with antiplatelet aggregation drugs initiated. It is not clear whether this approach effectively protects the patient against further neurological deterioration, but it might prevent further cardiac and cerebrovascular disease deterioration.

A trial of treatment with levodopa therapy is justified in all patients with VP, because there is no way to predict who will benefit. A substantial number of patients with clinically suspected VP respond to dopaminergic therapy, especially those with lesions in or close to the nigrostriatal pathway. The response to levodopa is not as remarkable as in patients with PD, and higher daily doses are needed; the dose of levodopa (with carbidopa) should be raised to 1500 mg/day before such treatment is considered a failure. Possible explanations for the positive levodopa response in patients with VP is the presence of a remaining pool of striatal dopaminergic nerve terminals in the dysfunctional nigrostriatal pathway that is sufficient to convert exogenous levodopa into dopamine and, thereby, to restore the intrinsic dopaminergic drive, or that the patient has coexisting VP and PD.

In patients with a dominant gait disorder, rehabilitation by a multidisciplinary team is highly important. Some patients benefit from the use of visual cues, e.g. walking with upturned walking sticks. Many patients are limited by fear of falling, and can be helped with behavior modification therapy.

Conclusion

Vascular parkinsonism is a heterogeneous disorder. The diagnosis should not be based on clinical grounds alone, and must also include the evaluation of risk factors, routine brain imaging, and nuclear imaging of the pre- and post-synaptic dopaminergic components. Together, these will maximize the accuracy of the diagnosis and will assist the clinician in tailoring treatment to the individual patient and also in giving advice on the progression and prognosis of the disease.

Ruth Djaldetti, Eldad Melamed

References

1 Foltynie T, Barker R, Brayne C. Vascular parkinsonism: a review of the precision and frequency of the diagnosis. *Neuroepidemiology* 2002; **21**: 1–7.

2 Hughes AJ, Daniel SE, Kilford L, Lees AJ. Accuracy of clinical diagnosis of idiopathic Parkinson's disease: a clinico-pathological study of 100 cases. *J Neurol Neurosurg Psychiatry* 1992; **55**: 181–4.

3 Rampello L, Alvano A, Battaglia G, Raffaele R, Vecchio I, Malaguarnera M. Different clinical and evolutional patterns in late idiopathic and vascular parkinsonism. *J Neurol* 2005; **252**: 1045–9.

4 Winikates J, Jankovic J. Clinical correlates of vascular parkinsonism. *Arch Neurol* 1999; **56**: 98–102.

5 Bower JH, Dickson DW, Taylor L, Maraganore DM, Rocca WA. Clinical correlates of the pathology underlying parkinsonism: a population perspective. *Mov Disord* 2002; **17**: 910–16.

6 Zijlmans J, Daniel SE, Hughes AJ, Révész T, Lees AJ. Clinicopathological investigation of vascular parkinsonism, including clinical criteria for diagnosis. *Mov Disord* 2004; **19**: 630–40.

7 Yamanouchi H, Nagura H. Neurological signs and frontal white matter lesions in vascular parkinsonism: a clinicopathologic study. *Stroke* 1997; **28**: 965–9.

8 Jellinger KA. The neuropathologic diagnosis of secondary parkinsonian syndromes. In: Battistin L, Scarlato G, Caraceni T, Ruggieri S, eds. *Advanced Neurology,* Vol. 69. New York: Raven Press, 1996: 293–303.

9 Critchley M. Arteriosclerotic parkinsonism. *Brain* 1929; **52**: 23–83.

10 Zijlmans JCM, Thijssen HOM, Vogels OJM. MRI in patients with suspected VP. *Neurology* 1995; **45**: 2183–8.

11 Marshall V, Grossert D. Role of dopamine transporter imaging in routine clinical practice. *Mov Disord* 2003; **18**: 1415–23.

12 Zijlmans J, Evans A, Fontes F *et al.* [123I] FP-CIT SPECT study in vascular parkinsonism and Parkinson's disease. *Mov Disord* 2007; **22**(9): 1278–85.

13 Lorberboym M, Djaldetti R, Melamed E, Sadeh M, Lampl Y. ^{123}I-FP-CIT SPECT imaging of dopamine transporters in patients with cerebrovascular disease and clinical diagnosis of vascular parkinsonism. *J Nucl Med* 2004; **45**: 1688–93.

Case study 18

Case presentation

Mrs S., a 53-year-old female, was referred for psychiatric evaluation and treatment by her movement disorders neurologist for depressed mood. Mrs S. was first diagnosed with Parkinson's disease (PD) at age 51. She has no other active medical or neurological conditions, and her only medications are pramipexole 1 mg t.i.d. and several over-the-counter medications for constipation.

Mrs S. has a college education and has been married for 30 years. She has never smoked tobacco, rarely drinks alcohol, and has one cup of caffeinated coffee a day. There is no personal or family history of substance abuse or any other psychiatric disorder. She owns a small clothing store.

Mrs S. showed up for her initial psychiatric evaluation by herself, though she usually attended neurological appointments with her husband. At first, the patient focused on her depressive symptoms, including sad mood, loss of interest in previously pleasurable activities, feelings of guilt, hopelessness, and passive suicide ideation. She stated that these symptoms had been present for the past 2 years, that she had never felt this way before, and that she was not sure if there were any psychosocial factors that might be contributing to her depression. She denied any symptoms of mania/hypomania (e.g. elevated mood, grandiose thinking, decreased need for sleep, or rapid speech), psychosis, or cognitive impairment. She claimed that her PD symptoms were well managed and interfered minimally with her functioning. Mrs S. appeared somewhat guarded on interview, so the psychiatrist inquired about the state of her small business and her marriage. At this point the patient burst into tears and told the following story.

At the time of her PD diagnosis, the patient was started on pramipexole and coenzyme Q_{10}. She also briefly attended a PD support group, but did not find it helpful. The initial pramipexole dosage was 0.125 mg t.i.d., which was slowly increased to 1.0 mg t.i.d. over the course of 18 months. Approximately 4 months after starting PD pharmacotherapy, she started to frequent nearby casinos and gamble. Mrs S. soon thought about gambling constantly, had strong urges to gamble, and felt a lack of control over the thoughts, urges, and gambling behaviors. She felt that she had become a different person, and that her personality had changed somehow. Once the symptoms developed and she reported sadness and other depressive symptoms to her neurologist, she was started on fluoxetine 20 mg/day, but did not experience any benefit.

The gambling behaviors steadily worsened over the next 18 months. Mrs S. ultimately lost approximately $500 000 and was forced to declare bankruptcy. During this period, to maintain her gambling behavior, she stole money from her husband and friends, and frequently lied to continue gambling.

When Mrs S. was asked during the initial interview why she did not inform her neurologist about her compulsive gambling, she stated that she was very ashamed of her behavior, and did not see how they were relevant to her PD.

Differential diagnosis

Multiple terms have been used to describe the clinical presentation of impulsive and compulsive behaviors in PD. Most behaviors described in PD have both impulsive (lack of forethought or consideration of consequences) and compulsive (repetitious behaviors with a lack of self-control) aspects. Impulse control disorders (ICDs) constitute a group of psychiatric disorders in the Diagnostic and Statistical Manual of Mental Disorders (DSM-IV-TR), and are characterized by a failure to resist an impulse, drive, or temptation to perform a typically pleasurable activity that is ultimately harmful to the person or to others owing to its excessive nature. Pathological or compulsive gambling is the most common ICD, and other ICDs without formal DSM-IV-TR diagnostic criteria include compulsive sexual behavior and compulsive buying. Binge eating disorder, classified as an eating disorder in the DSM-IV-TR, shares many of the clinical features of ICDs.

Also reported to occur in PD is punding, non-pleasurable and non-harmful compulsive behaviors characterized by complex, prolonged, purposeless, and stereotyped acts (e.g. fascination with manipulating small objects) [1]. A related disorder, termed walkabout, is characterized by excessive, aimless walking or driving. Thus, ICDs may represent the severe end of a spectrum of behavioral disturbances in PD that are characterized by poorly controlled repetitive behaviors.

The terms dopamine dysregulation syndrome (DDS), hedonistic homeostatic dysregulation, dopamimetic drug addiction, and compulsive dopaminergic drug use have been used to describe a syndrome in which patients increase on their own or take excessively large amounts of their PD medications, typically shorter-acting drugs such as levodopa or subcutaneous apomorphine. Patients with DDS typically develop cyclical mood disorders (i.e. mood elevation or hypomania secondary to dopamine replacement therapy use, followed by a dysphoric affective state when medications are withdrawn or reduced). When in an elevated state, patients may be excessively involved in pleasurable activities that have a high potential for painful consequences [2].

This syndrome seems distinct from ICDs in many ways, as few PD patients with an ICD are reported either to compulsively use their PD medications or to experience mood elevation, and many patients with DDS do not have a comorbid ICD [3].

Other psychiatric disorders or behaviors that share features of ICDs have been reported to occur in PD. For instance, obsessive-compulsive disorder (OCD), an anxiety disorder characterized by the repetition of non-pleasurable, non-harmful behaviors (e.g. checking or counting) to reduce anxiety, may occur at an increased frequency in PD, although it has not been reported in association with PD medications. It is important to note that the types of impulsive and compulsive behaviors previously described also do not occur in the context of obsessive-compulsive *personality* disorder, a lifelong personality style characterized by preoccupation with orderliness, perfectionism, and control.

Case diagnosis and treatment

At the conclusion of the initial evaluation, the psychiatrist called the neurologist and informed him of Mrs S.'s diagnoses of an ICD (i.e. compulsive gambling) and a depressive disorder secondary to the ICD. She did not have mood, cognitive, or behavioral changes consistent either with a manic episode or DDS secondary to overuse of PD medications. A decision was made to quickly taper and discontinue pramipexole treatment, substituting levodopa for the management of PD symptoms. As part of treatment cross-titration, controlled-release levodopa was initiated at 25/100 b.i.d. At her next office visit, Mrs S. reported that all thoughts and urges to gamble, as well as all gambling behaviors, were completely resolved within 1 month of pramipexole discontinuation. At a subsequent psychiatric appointment, the patient volunteered that she had also experienced compulsive eating behaviors, including a new-onset craving for sweets with a resultant 15 kg weight gain, in the context of pramipexole treatment. These symptoms also resolved with the change to levodopa.

Five years later, Mrs S. was taking carbidopa 37.5 mg/levodopa 150 mg/entacapone 200 mg b.i.d. and no other PD medications. Over this time period, she was also prescribed several antidepressants, including escitalopram and bupropion, for chronic depressive symptoms, but did not experience any benefit. She eventually had to sell her business, and her husband divorced her. Though she had not gambled in the 5 years since stopping pramipexole treatment, Mrs S. stated that her life had been irreparably damaged by her gambling behavior.

Final diagnosis: treatment-related impulse control disorder.

Discussion

Overview of ICDs in PD

Retrospective and prospective case reporting have indicated compulsive gambling rates of 0.5–4.4% in PD [4,5], and a cumulative incidence rate of 2.4% was reported for compulsive sexual behavior [6]. Compulsive eating has been reported in PD, but its prevalence is not known [2,7]. In two recent large-scale screening studies, a frequency of 1.7% for compulsive gambling was reported in one [8], and the frequency of at least one active ICD (compulsive gambling, sexual behavior, or buying) was 4.0% in the other [9]. In the latter study, compulsive sexual behavior was as common as problem gambling (2.6% vs. 2.2%, respectively), and the frequency of compulsive buying was 0.4%. Though finding an appropriate comparison group is difficult, a recent study found that PD patients were approximately 25 times more likely to have compulsive gambling than an age- and sex-matched control group [10].

Case reporting has implicated dopamine agonists (DAs), and much less commonly levodopa, as precipitating compulsive gambling [4,5] and sexual behavior [11] in PD. In one of the aforementioned screening studies [8], compulsive gambling was significantly more common in DA-treated patients than in those on levodopa monotherapy, and in the other study [9], all active ICD cases were currently taking a DA, with no differences in ICD frequency for the three DAs examined (pramipexole, ropinirole, and pergolide). Thus, the pharmacotherapy risk associated with ICDs seems specific to the DA medication class, and perhaps greatest at dosages at the high end of the therapeutic range [3,9].

Looking at other potential risk factors, PD patients with ICDs have disproportionately been younger males in case reporting [11]. In one of the aforementioned screening studies [9], a history of ICD symptomatology prior to PD was the only significant predictor (other than DA use) of an ICD using multivariate analysis. In the other study [8], compulsive gambling was associated with earlier PD onset, and the majority of these patients had either a premorbid personal or family history of alcohol use disorder, or a family history of bipolar disorder. Similarly, in a study of DDS in PD, patients with DDS (over half of whom had comorbid ICDs) had younger age of PD onset and were more likely to have a past history of substance abuse [12].

Although the neurobiology of ICDs in PD is not well understood, the pronounced depletion of dopamine in the nigrostriatal pathway (leading to disruption in cortical–subcortical circuitry) is thought to contribute to the development of numerous psychiatric and cognitive disorders in PD. Second, PD patients, even those without dementia, commonly display impairment in executive abilities, and executive impairments such as poor decision-making and response inhibition are thought to contribute to the development of ICDs. Finally, DAs compared with levodopa have significantly higher D_3: D_2 and D_3: D_1 striatal receptor activation ratios. The D_3 receptor is concentrated in limbic areas of the brain, including the ventral striatum, and may mediate psychiatric manifestations of dopamine receptor stimulation.

Clinically, the apparent under-recognition of ICDs in PD should be addressed through a careful history and patient education prior to initiating DA treatment, and by regular monitoring for ICDs throughout the course of treatment. If a clinician suspects the presence of an ICD and needs assistance in the assessment and management process, then the patient should be promptly referred to a psychiatrist for a comprehensive evaluation and ongoing care.

Regarding the neurological management of ICDs, case reporting and anecdotal experience suggest that ICD behaviors often resolve after reducing the dose of the existing DA, switching to a different DA, discontinuing DA treatment entirely, or perhaps receiving counseling [4,13]. Although ICDs may worsen transiently immediately after subthalamic nucleus (STN) deep brain stimulation (DBS), chronic STN DBS is associated with improvement in ICD symptoms, perhaps secondary to an overall reduction in PD pharmacotherapy postsurgery [14].

A range of psychiatric pharmacological treatments, most commonly selective serotonin reuptake inhibitors, have been used in the treatment of ICDs in PD, but there is no empirical evidence to support their use for this indication in PD. There are also individual case reports of successful treatment of compulsive gambling in PD with either risperidone or quetiapine. Regarding nonpharmacological approaches, behavioral treatments (e.g. cognitive behavioral therapy) and attendance at self-help groups have not been formally examined for the treatment of ICDs in PD.

Daniel Weintraub

References

1 Miyasaki J, Hassan KL, Lang AE *et al*. Punding prevalence in Parkinson's disease. *Mov Disord* 2007; **22**: 1179–81.

2 Giovannoni G, O'Sullivan JD, Turner K *et al*. Hedonistic homeostatic dysregulation in patients with Parkinson's disease on dopamine replacement therapies. *J Neurol Neurosurg Psychiatry* 2000; 68: 423–8.

3 Gallagher DA, O'Sullivan SS, Evans AH *et al*. Pathological gambling in Parkinson's disease: risk factors and differences from dopamine dysregulation. An analysis of published case series. *Mov Disord* 2007; **22**(12): 1757–63.

4 Driver-Dunckley E, Samanta J, Stacy M. Pathological gambling associated with dopamine agonist therapy in Parkinson's disease. *Neurology* 2003; **61**: 422–3.

5 Grosset KA, Macphee G, Pal G *et al*. Problematic gambling on dopamine agonists: not such a rarity. *Mov Disord* 2006; **21**(12): 2206–8.

6 Voon V, Hassan K, Zurowski M *et al*. Prevalence of repetitive and reward-seeking behaviors in Parkinson disease. *Neurology* 2006; **67**: 1254–7.

7 Nirenberg MJ, Waters C. Compulsive eating and weight gain related to dopamine agonist use. *Mov Disord* 2006; **21**(4): 524–9.

8 Voon V, Hassan K, Zurowski M *et al*. Prospective prevalence of pathological gambling and medication association in Parkinson disease. *Neurology* 2006; **66**: 1750–2.

9 Weintraub D, Siderowf AD, Potenza MN *et al*. Association of dopamine agonist use with impulse control disorders in Parkinson disease. *Arch Neurol* 2006; **63**: 969–73.

10 Avanzi M, Baratti M, Cabrini S *et al*. Prevalence of pathological gambling in patients with Parkinson's disease. *Mov Disord* 2006; **21**(12): 2068–72.

11 Klos KJ, Bower JH, Josephs KA *et al.* Pathological hypersexuality predominantly linked to adjuvant dopamine agonist therapy in Parkinson's disease and multiple system atrophy. *Parkinsonism Relat Disord* 2005; **11**(6): 381–6.

12 Evans AH, Lawrence AD, Potts J *et al.* Factors influencing susceptibility to compulsive dopaminergic drug use in Parkinson disease. *Neurology* 2005; **65**: 1570–4.

13 Mamikonyan E, Siderowf AD, Duda JE *et al.* Long-term follow-up of impulse control disorders in Parkinson's disease. *Mov Disord* 2007; Oct 25 [Epub ahead of print].

14 Ardouin C, Voon V, Worbe Y *et al.* Pathological gambling in Parkinson's disease improves on chronic subthalamic nucleus stimulation. *Mov Disord* 2006; **21**(11): 1941–6.

Case study 19

Case presentation

This 61-year-old man of French ancestry was born to non-consanguineous parents and had no personal or familial medical history. He had three children and worked as a garage foreman. At the age of 57 years, he first noticed difficulties in walking and in moving his left arm. Neurological examination disclosed asymmetric akinesia and rigidity on his left side and a treatment with levodopa was introduced. No resting tremor was noticed. The Unified Parkinson's Disease Rating Scale (UPDRS) total motor score dropped from 26 before levodopa treatment to 5 a few months later.

The patient was first seen in our department when 60 years old. At that time, he was treated with levodopa/benserazide (800 mg/200 mg/day) in four divided doses. He complained of diminished levodopa effectiveness. Examination showed severe bilateral akinesia and rigidity predominating in upper and lower left limbs, walking problems, and no resting tremor. The UPDRS motor score before and 40 min after a single dose of levodopa/benserazide (200 mg/50 mg) dropped from 40 to 28 (30% improvement). Mild dyskinesias consisting in right foot dystonia followed by trunk and upper limb choreic movements were noticed during the test. There was no orthostatic hypotension.

In addition to parkinsonism, the patient had marked cognitive problems. Mini Mental Status Examination (MMSE) was 21/30, the Frontal Assessment Battery (FAB) was 10/18, and the Mattis Dementia Rating Scale (MDRS) was 117/144. Working memory was impaired as well as clock drawing, suggesting constructional apraxia. Bilateral gestural apraxia was also noticed.

Brain magnetic resonance imaging (MRI) was normal, but scintigraphy with technetium-99m ethyl cysteinate dimer (^{99m}Tc ECD) single photon emission computed tomography (SPECT) showed decreased perfusion of the prefrontal, parietal, and temporal cortex bilaterally. Positron emission tomography (PET) scan with [^{18}F]fluoro-L-dopa revealed bilateral decreased binding of the marker in posterior thirds of putamina and to a lesser extent in both heads of the caudate nuclei. Striatal binding of [^{11}C]raclopride, a high-affinity D2 dopamine receptor antagonist, was slightly decreased compared to control patients.

Systematic blood analysis was unremarkable, except for the presence of mild thrombocytopenia (around 100 000 platelets/mm^3).

Differential diagnosis

Parkinsonism was initially unremarkable in our patient. Although there was no resting tremor, akinesia and rigidity were asymmetric, and responded well to levodopa, suggesting sporadic Parkinson's disease (PD). Age at onset was in the expected range for PD and the presence of levodopa-induced dyskinesia was also in line with this diagnosis. There were, however, several atypical features. First, reactivity to levodopa progressively diminished with only 30% reactivity after 3 years. Second, the patient exhibited severe cognitive problems early within the disease course and at a relatively young age, together with signs of cortical involvement such as constructional and gestural apraxia and diffuse cortical hypoperfusion.

At the same time, the discovery of a thrombocytopenia led to further explorations that revealed splenomegaly and high ferritin levels. A bone marrow biopsy analysis showed the presence of lipid-laden macrophages suggesting Gaucher disease (GD). Glucocerebrosidase activity was very low (10% of the normal value) and the patient was shown to be homozygote for the N370S mutation, confirming GD. Further investigations did not reveal any osseous involvement. Given the mild systemic involvement and the presence of rapidly progressive parkinsonism and dementia, miglustat was introduced (100 mg t.i.d). After 12 months, however, cognitive function continued to deteriorate. An acute therapeutic test with levodopa/benserazide (200 mg/50 mg) showed weak levodopa responsiveness: the UPDRS motor score dropped from 36 before treatment to 32. Cognitive problems had also worsened: MMSE was 19/30, FAB was 4/18 and MDRS was 94/144. Treatment with miglustat was interrupted because of the lack of efficacy on neurological progression and because GD was mild not necessitating treatment.

Final diagnosis: Gaucher disease complicated by parkinsonism.

Discussion

Gaucher disease and parkinsonism

GD is the most prevalent inherited lysosomal storage disorder. It is caused by a recessively inherited deficiency of glucocerebrosidase (GBA). The enzymatic block results in the accumulation of glucocerebrosides mainly in macrophage lysosomes.

GD is classified into three types based on age at onset, disease course, and the presence or absence of neurological signs. GD type 1 is the most common variant (around 95% of cases). Clinical symptoms appear at any age from childhood to adulthood, and usually include hepatosplenomegaly, thrombo-cytopenia, pancytopenia, bleeding, and osseous manifestations (pain and fractures). The course is chronic and, by definition, nervous system involve-ment is absent. Some patients with GD type 1 remain virtually asymptom-atic, being diagnosed during evaluation for a non-related disorder or familial screening of a symptomatic relative. GD type 2 is an acute "neuronopathic" disease which begins in early infancy and usually leads to death within the first 2 years of life because of severe neurological signs. Type 3 is intermedi-ate between types 2 and 1. It can begin at any age between childhood and adulthood, displays a chronic course, and involves the nervous system in ad-dition to systemic signs. Characteristic neurological signs include horizontal oculomotor apraxia which can remain isolated, myoclonic epilepsy, cerebellar ataxia, dystonia, pyramidal signs, and extrapyramidal signs.

This classification has been questioned in recent years, however, with the observations that some patients with GD type 1 do occasionally develop par-kinsonism and that specific brain lesions may be observed independently of the presence or absence of neurological symptoms. These observations sug-gest a continuum between neuronopathic and non-neuronopathic forms of GD.

From the analysis of 32 patients previously reported in the literature as well as 5 patients in our unit, the specificity of parkinsonism in patients with GD type 1 can be defined as follows [1,2]:

• *Frequency of PD in GD*: Bembi *et al.* [3] found 4 patients with parkinsonism in a series of 58 GD patients (6.9%). Neudorfer *et al.* [4] found 3 patients with PD in a series of 130 patients (2.3%). Thus the prevalence of PD seems at least 10 times higher in GD patients than in the general population (0.1% under the age of 65 years).

• *Age at onset of PD in GD*: Mean age of onset of parkinsonism is 49 years in GD. This is 10 years earlier than in sporadic PD where the median age at onset is 60 or more.

• *Clinical characteristics of PD in GD*: Among 32 patients with PD and GD on whom data is available, sustained response to levodopa has been reported in only 5 patients (16%), whereas other patients exhibited no response, partial response or transient response (as in our patient). Atypical signs usually ab-sent in PD have occasionally been observed, including perception deafness (2 patients), horizontal oculomotor apraxia (2 patients), myoclonus (2 patients) or dementia (7 patients).

• *Neuropathological abnormalities in patients with GD and PD*: Eight patients with GD and PD have been studied at the neuropathological level by Wong *et al.* [5] and Tayebi *et al.* [6]. All exhibited neuronal loss and Lewy bodies in the sub-stantia nigra. In addition, 5 patients among 8 (62.5%) presented diffuse Lewy bodies in hippocampal CA2–4 neurons, a feature usually not seen in PD but characteristic of dementia with Lewy bodies (DLB). Furthermore, Wong *et al.* reported astrogliosis of laminae 3, 4b, and 5 of the cortex and in the hippocam-pal CA2 region, which is also a frequent feature in DLB.

• *Treatment of patients with PD and GD*: Although systemic manifestations of GD do respond to enzyme replacement therapy, no effect was noticed on parkinsonism in all 12 patients reported with GD and PD treated with this therapy (which does not cross the brain barrier). Miglustat, an *N*-alkylated imino sugar that inhibits glucocerebroside synthesis and could in theory cross the blood–brain barrier, should be more efficacious. Only one report, however, has claimed some stabilization of parkinsonism with this treatment. We have treated two patients with GD and PD for 12 months: one of the patients seems to be stable now; the other (presented here) clearly has some worsening of dementia and weaker levodopa responsiveness.

• *Mutations of GBA in PD and DLB*: Interestingly, mutations in the gene coding for *GBA* have frequently been found in patients with sporadic PD, suggesting that *GBA* mutations even in heterozygotes constitute a contributing risk factor for PD. In a first postmortem study from North America, 8 patients with mutations in the *GBA* gene were discovered among 57 PD patients (14%) as opposed to zero mutations in 44 control brains [7]. In most cases, mutations were in the heterozygous state; but in two cases, mutations were homozygote. These results have been reproduced in different populations including Ashkenazi Jews where the frequency of heterozygotes is around 5–10 times higher (31% mutations among 99 PD patients against 6.2% in 1543 controls, and 4.1% in 74 patients with Alzheimer disease); Canadians (10.7% N370S mutation among 160 PD patients against 4.3% in 92 controls), Venezuelans (12% mutations among 33 PD patients against 3% in 31 controls) and Taiwanese (4.3% mutations among 92 PD patients against 1.1% in 92 controls). The only negative study was in the Norwegian population where no difference was found between patients with PD and controls. Overall, these independent studies have demonstrated a statistical association between PD and mutations in the *GBA* gene. Papers are conflicting regarding whether PD in heretozygotes for the *GBA* mutation is different from idiopathic PD. In the largest series, no difference was found with respect to age at onset, type of symptoms, or levodopa response. Recently, however, it has been shown that heterozygotes were even more frequent among patients with DLB (23% mutations among 35 patients with DLB as opposed to zero mutations in 12 subjects with multiple system atrophy and only 4% in 28 patients with PD [8]).

• *Pathophysiology*: The link between glucocerebrosidase gene mutations and PD is not well understood. Glucocerebroside accumulation could have an excitotoxic effect by activation of ryanodin receptors that would in turn provoke the release of endogenous calcium from the endoplasmic reticulum. Another hypothesis comes from the observation that glucocerebrosides recognize α-synuclein and could therefore facilitate fibrillization of the protein in neurons, a process known to play a role in the pathology of PD and DLB. Observations that PD (and DLB) is observed with mutations in GBA both in heterozygotes and in homozygotes and that no glucocerebroside accumulation has been demonstrated in these patients, however, challenge these hypotheses. A recently favored hypothesis is that mutated *GBA* could have an abnormal conformation that interferes with chaperone-mediated autophagy of synuclein inside the lysosome. In favor of this "gain of function hypothesis," all *GBA* mutations found so far in subjects with PD or DLB are missense mutations that could potentially change the conformation of the protein.

Parkinsonism and inherited metabolic diseases

Parkinsonism can be found in numerous inherited metabolic diseases including metal storage disorders (Wilson's disease, hemochromatosis, aceruloplasminemia, neuroferritinopathy), various mitochondrial cytopathies (polymerase gamma mutations, leber mutations, complex 1 deficiency, Twinkle mutations, etc.), lysosomal storage disorders (ceroid lipofuscinoses, GM1 and GM2 gangliosidosis, Niemann-Pick disease type C), dopamine synthesis defects (Segawa disease and related disorders), and miscellaneous disorders (polyglucosan body diseases, cerebrotendinous xanthomatosis, homocystinuria) (see Table 3.19.1). In most cases, typical features on brain MRI or associated clinical signs easily distinguish inherited metabolic diseases from PD. To our knowledge, among inherited metabolic diseases, isolated PD has only been observed in certain mitochondrial disorders, pyruvate dehydrogenase deficiency, hemochromatosis, phenylketonuria, guanosine 5'-triphosphate cyclohydrolase (GTPC) 1 deficiency, Wilson's disease, and GD. DLB-like phenotype has only been reported in GD [9].

Frédéric Sedel

References

1 Cherin P, Sedel F, Mignot C et al. Neurological manifestations of type 1 Gaucher's disease: is a revision of disease classification needed? *Rev Neurol* 2006; **162**: 1076–83.
2 Sidransky E. Gaucher disease and parkinsonism. *Mol Genet Metab* 2005; **84**: 302–4.
3 Bembi B, Zambito Marsala S, Sidransky E et al. GD's disease with Parkinson's disease: clinical and pathological aspects. *Neurology* 2003; **61**: 99–101.
4 Neudorfer O, Giladi N, Elstein D et al. Occurrence of Parkinson's syndrome in type I GD. *QJM.* 1996; **89**: 691–4.
5 Wong K, Sidransky E, Verma A et al. Neuropathology provides clues to the pathophysiology of GD. *Mol Genet Metab* 2004; **82**: 192–207.
6 Tayebi N, Walker J, Stubblefield B et al. GD with parkinsonian manifestations: does glucocerebrosidase deficiency contribute to a vulnerability to parkinsonism? *Mol Genet Metab* 2003; **79**: 104–9.
7 Lwin A, Orvisky E, Goker-Alpan O, LaMarca ME, Sidransky E. Glucocerebrosidase mutations in subjects with parkinsonism. *Mol Genet Metab* 2004; **81**: 70–3.
8 Hruska KS, Goker-Alpan O, Sidransky E. Gaucher disease and the synucleinopathies. *J Biomed Biotechnol* 2006; **3**: 78549.
9 Sedel F, Lyon-Caen O, Saudubray JM. Therapy insight: inborn errors of metabolism in adult neurology – a clinical approach focused on treatable diseases. *Nat Clin Pract Neurol* 2007; **3**(5): 279–90.

Table 3.19.1 Parkinsonism in adult patients with inborn errors of metabolism

Disease	Mode of inheritance	Age at onset (years)[a]	Major clinical and radiological signs other than parkinsonism that can be found in adults	Major biological disturbances	Treatment	Response to levodopa[b]
Metal storage disorders						
Wilson's disease	AR	55	Psychiatric signs, action tremor, dystonia, dysarthria, Kayser–Fleischer ring, chronic liver disease. High signal of basal ganglia (thalami, putamina), dentate nuclei, brainstem white matter on T2-weighted sequences	High urinary copper, low plasma copper and ceruloplasmin	D-penicillamine, zinc, trientine	–
Hemochromatosis	AR	> 50	Cerebellar ataxia, dementia, myoclonus, action tremor, dystonia, pyramidal syndrome, liver complications, arthritis, endocrinopathy, cardiomyopathy, bronze skin pigmentation, and asthenia. Normal MRI or brain atrophy	High levels of serum iron, transferrin saturation, and ferritin. Search for C282Y mutation in the HFE gene	Phlebotomy (not efficient on parkinsonism)	+
Aceruloplasminemia	AR		Chorea, dystonia, dementia, diabetes, retinal degeneration. Brain MRI: low signal intensity (iron deposits) putamina, caudate, thalami, dentate nuclei	Low levels of serum ceruloplasmin, copper, iron High levels of ferritin Microcytic anemia Mutations in the ceruloplasmin gene	Iron chelators?	–
Neuroferritinopathy	AD	> 50	Chorea, dystonia, dysarthria. Brain MRI: low signal intensity (iron deposits) in red nuclei, putamina, caudate, pallidum, substantia nigra, thalami, bipallidal hyperintensities or necrosis	Low levels of serum ferritin FTL1 mutations (ferritin light chain polypeptide)	Iron chelators?	–

Lysosomal storage diseases

Kufs' disease	Sporadic, AR and AD	> 50	Type A: progressive myoclonic epilepsy; Type B: movement disorders, dementia, cerebellar ataxia	Intraneuronal autofluorescent inclusions: fingerprint profiles or granular osmiophilic deposits by electron microscopy of skin, rectal or brain biopsy	Symptomatic	–
CLN3	AR	10	Retinitis pigmentosa, generalized epilepsy, ataxia, cognitive troubles	Mutations in the CLN3 (Battenin) gene	Symptomatic	+
Gaucher disease	AR	> 50	Dementia, progressive myoclonic epilepsy, supranuclear ophthalmoplegia (horizontal), ataxia, asthenia, splenomegaly, hepatomegaly, thrombopenia, anemia, osseous manifestations	Low glucocerebrosidase activity	Enzymotherapy	+
GM2 gangliosidosis (adult form)	AR	35	Cerebellar ataxia, pyramidal signs, psychiatric troubles, lower motor neuron disease, sensory polyneuropathy, dystonia	Low hexosaminidases activity in leukocytes	None (miglustat?)	–
Niemann-Pick disease type C	AR	> 50	Vertical oculomotor apraxia, cerebellar ataxia, psychiatric signs, dementia, dystonia, splenomegaly, hepatomegaly	Abnormal filipin staining of fibroblasts (accumulation of free cholesterol in lysosomes)	Miglustat?	–
GM1 gangliosidosis	AR	20	Generalized dystonia, dysarthria, kyphoscoliosis, vertebral and hip dysplasia	Low β-galactosidase activity in leukocytes	Miglustat?	–

(Continued.)

Table 3.19.1 (Continued.)

Disease	Mode of inheritance	Age at onset (years)[a]	Major clinical and radiological signs other than parkinsonism that can be found in adults	Major biological disturbances	Treatment	Response to levodopa[b]
Energy metabolism defects						
Pyruvate dehydrogenase (PDH) deficiency	X linked or AR	50	Acute signs: ataxia, dystonia, weakness, confusion, coma, oculomotor palsies Chronic signs: dystonia Brain MRI: normal or bilateral putaminal necrosis (Leigh syndrome)	High postprandial lactate (L) and pyruvate (P) with L/P ratio<20, low PDH activity (fibroblasts)	Thiamine, ketogenic diet	–
Respiratory chain disorders	Any	> 50	Progressive external ophthalmoplegia, myopathy, hearing loss, cerebellar ataxia, retinitis pigmentosa, stroke-like episodes, diabetes, polyneuropathy	High lactate in CSF, ragged red fibers (muscular biopsy), analysis of respiratory chain activity (muscle biopsy), search for mitochondrial or nuclear DNA specific mutations	None	+
Dopamine synthesis defects						
GTP cyclohydrolase 1 deficiency	AD	> 50	Dystonia (may mimic spastic paraparesis), diurnal fluctuations	Mutations in the GTPCH1 gene, low biopterins, neopterins, HVA and 5HIAA in CSF.	Levodopa, anticholinergic drugs, dopamine agonists	++
Other dopamine synthesis defects	AR	< 10	Dystonia, mental retardation, hypersomnolence, pyramidal signs, epilepsy, oculogyric crisis.	Low HVA in CSF, other abnormalities depend on the metabolic block	Levodopa, 5-hydroxy tryptophan, BH4 (depending on the metabolic defect)	++

Miscellaneous disorders

Disease	Inheritance	Max age of onset[a]	Clinical features	Biochemical findings	Treatment	Response[b]
Polyglucosan body disease	AR	> 50	Dementia, upper and lower motor neuron disease, bladder dysfunction, leukodystrophy	Evidence of polyglucosan bodies on axillary biopsy	None	–
Cerebrotendinous xanthomatosis	AR	> 50	Juvenile cataract, xanthomas, cerebellar ataxia, spastic paraparesis, dementia, psychiatric signs, parkinsonism, chronic diarrhea	High cholestanol and sterol intermediates	Chenodeoxycholic acid	+
Phenylketonuria	AR	45	Optic atrophy, dementia, leukoencephalopathy, parkinsonism	Hyperphenylalaninemia, hypotyrosinemia	Poor phenylalanine diet	++
Cystathionine β-synthase deficiency	AR	50	Mental retardation, disorders of personality or behavior. Rare cases of psychosis. Epilepsy, strokes, dystonia, thromboembolic events, marfan-like appearance, lens dislocation.	Hyperhomocysteinemia, >100µM, hypermethioninemia	Vitamin B6+/- low methionine diet	–

[a] Maximum age of onset, based on literature review or on author's own experience.
[b] –, no response, +, partial, transient or not always responsive, ++, good response.

Case presentation

A 76-year-old farmer with primary-school education was referred to the clinic for slowness of movement, apathy, and mental dysfunction.

The history revealed that his complaints had started gradually 3 years previously. His initial symptoms were slowing of walking with short steps and general slowing of body movements, soon followed by a resting tremor of the right hand. He was diagnosed as having Parkinson's disease (PD). Treatment with levodopa was initiated. Response was moderate but clear, so the treatment was maintained. Within the 6 months prior to the referral, new symptoms had emerged: he developed excessive daytime sleepiness and there were brief episodes of confusion with disorientation to place on awakening. He also became forgetful, sometimes had difficulties finding his way or the right room in his home, and his speech became increasingly slurred. At that time, he did not suffer from hallucinations, delusions, or aggression. His wife mentioned that he spoke and moved during his sleep, something which had developed over the previous 3–4 years. In the last few months, he developed urinary urgency and occasional incontinence.

His past medical history included long-standing hypertension. In the family history, his mother was said to have been forgetful in the later years of her life.

The neurological examination revealed bradymimia with masked facies, moderate hypophonia, and dysarthria with brisk nasopalpebral reflex. Eye movements were normal and the rest of the cranial nerves were inconspicuous. There was moderate bradykinesia and rigidity on both upper and lower extremities, with slow and irregular finger and foot-taps that were more prominent on the right side. Muscle tendon reflexes were symmetrical and normal; plantar reflexes were flexor; muscle strength and sensory examination were normal; and there were no cerebellar signs. Gait was slow and short stepped with reduced arm swing and occasional festination, especially when turning around. The pull test was normal with no signs of retropulsion.

In neuropsychological examination, he was cooperative with preserved insight into his mental difficulties. He was moderately apathetic and slow in responding. Attention was clearly impaired. He was unable to perform subtraction of serial sevens from 100 or recite the months of the years backwards. He recited the days of the week backwards with difficulty and frequent pauses. Memory testing revealed primarily retrieval deficits. After three encoding trials, he was able to remember one of three words in delayed free recall, remembered another one after cueing, and correctly identified the third one in recognition testing. His incidental memory was largely preserved; he was able to remember recent events and merely missed some details. Executive functions were clearly impaired: in verbal fluency testing, he was able to produce six words beginning with the letter A, four words with S, and name seven animals within one minute. The clock-drawing test revealed planning errors (Figure 3.20.1), there were slight problems with response inhibition in go/no-go test, and in the Trails B test, he had problems switching the strategy. Visuospatial functions were also significantly impaired. He was unable to copy intersecting pentagons or a three-dimensional cube, and could not imitate intercalating fingers with his hands. Core language functions and ideomotor praxis were intact.

Laboratory screening tests, including thyroid hormones, vitamin B12 levels and VDRL, were normal. Brain magnetic resonance imaging revealed mild atrophy, predominantly in frontal, and medial temporal areas and more so in parieto-occipital areas.

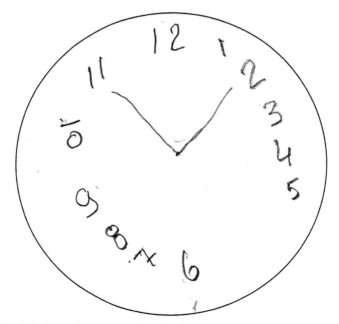

Figure 3.20.1 A clock-drawing test revealing planning errors.

Following the first examination, levodopa dose was increased to 125 mg levodopa/carbidopa q.i.d., and modafinil was added for daytime sleepiness. With this treatment, his gait and slowness of movements improved slightly, and daytime sleepiness was reduced. The patient developed vivid hallucinations, however, seeing children, old people, and animals. His confusion worsened, especially at night, and dream-enacting behavior became more prominent with frequent sleep interruptions. He was frequently disoriented to place, confusing his home and rooms, at times having blank stares, and not recognizing family members. He was no longer able to function independently and became increasingly dependent on his family for activities of daily living. A treatment with the cholinesterase inhibitor rivastigmine was initiated and titrated up to 4.5 mg b.i.d., and up to 2 mg of clonazepam was added for dream-enacting behavior. Following this treatment, the patient became more attentive, his confusion lessened, hallucinations and dream-enacting behavior improved, but his movements remained unchanged.

During further follow-up over 2 years, there was a slight decline from initial improvement in cognition, with occasional confusional episodes, hallucinations and misperceptions occurring occasionally. His speech gradually worsened with occasional difficulties in swallowing. His axial symptoms, notably initiation and turning difficulties, also got slightly worse. Levodopa was increased to 250 mg q.i.d. and rivastigmine to 6 mg b.i.d. during this period. The patient remained stable over the next 6 months.

Differential diagnosis

This patient initially developed a movement disorder with slowing of gait, bradykinesia, rigidity, and tremor with an asymmetrical onset. His symptoms were responsive to dopaminergic treatment. Within 2.5 years of disease onset, cognitive and behavioral symptoms emerged with increased daytime sleepiness, mental slowing, apathy, forgetfulness, visuospatial disorientation, delusions, and hallucinations with a gradual onset and successive worsening. These symptoms improved moderately upon treatment with a cholinesterase inhibitor. The further course was of a slight decline, both in motor (notably speech and other axial symptoms) and cognitive functions over 2 years.

Based on the initial symptoms a diagnosis of PD was made. There were no atypical or additional features that would suggest another form of parkinsonism. There were no cerebellar features or prominent autonomic symptoms reminiscent of multiple system atrophy (MSA). Eye movements were preserved making progressive supranuclear palsy (PSP) unlikely. Furthermore, early mental dysfunction, prominent asymmetry, apraxia, and dystonic features, which would raise the possibility of corticobasal ganglionic degeneration (CBGD), were also absent. The gradual onset and presence of an asymmetrical tremor are not typical for vascular parkinsonism, and brain imaging did not show any relevant vascular lesions. Likewise the history did not reveal any features suggestive of a symptomatic form such as neuroleptic-induced parkinsonism. Good response to levodopa also suggested that the initial diagnosis of PD was justified.

The emergence of cognitive dysfunction and behavioral symptoms within 2.5 years of disease onset is the key diagnostic feature in this patient. As in all cases where dementia is suspected, the diagnosis involves two steps. The first is to exclude other conditions associated with mental dysfunction which can mimic dementia, such as acute confusion (delirium) and depression. Confusion can be excluded, as mental dysfunction had an insidious onset and showed progressive worsening. Likewise depression is unlikely to be the cause of mental dysfunction because of the broad spectrum and profile of cognitive and behavioral symptoms, including visuospatial dysfunction and psychotic features. Based on the history and results of the neuropsychological examination, which revealed impairment in multiple cognitive domains and significant functional impairment, the diagnosis of a dementia syndrome is justified in this patient.

The differential diagnosis then includes all diseases that can present with a combination of parkinsonism and dementia. Dementia with Lewy bodies (DLB) is one of the most frequent of these conditions. This is, however, unlikely as the diagnostic criteria for DLB stipulate that motor and mental symptoms should start within 1 year of each other. Other neurodegenerative diseases, such as PSP or CBGD which present with combined motor–mental dysfunction, are also unlikely based on the clinical presentation. MSA can be associated with cognitive dysfunction; however, it is usually not as prominent as in this case. Other features typical of MSA were also missing. Coincident Alzheimer's disease (AD) can theoretically develop in a patient with PD; however, the profile of cognitive impairment in this patient was not that of AD, which is characterized by prominent and progressive amnesia as the core feature. Cerebrovascular disease can result in a combined motor–mental impairment, but this can be excluded based on history, the profile of parkinsonism, and the lack of vascular lesions in imaging. Likewise, normal pressure hydrocephalus, other symptomatic forms of parkinsonism associated with dementia, such as space-occupying lesions, and systemic diseases can be excluded based on imaging and laboratory findings. Central nervous system infections such as Creutzfeldt–Jakob disease are unlikely based on the disease course.

Given the initial, justified diagnosis of PD and later, gradual emergence of dementia 2.5 years after the disease onset, the most likely diagnosis in this patient is Parkinson's disease with dementia (PDD). The profile of cognitive symptoms with predominant impairment of attention, executive and visuospatial functions with less prominent amnesia, and multiple associated behavioral symptoms such as excessive daytime sleepiness, apathy, and hallucinations are typical for PDD. There are no auxiliary investigations to confirm the diagnosis. Imaging usually reveals mild atrophy predominantly in medial temporal, frontal, and especially in parieto-occipital areas, which was the case in this patient. The moderate response to cholinergic treatment is compatible with this diagnosis, as cholinesterase inhibitors have been shown to be of benefit in patients with PDD.

Final diagnosis: dementia associated with Parkinson's disease.

Discussion

Dementia affects 30–40% of all PD patients during the course of their disease; the incidence of dementia in PD is six times higher than in the general population. The clinical features of PDD are different than those seen in AD and can be summarized as a dysexecutive syndrome with impaired attention, executive dysfunction, early and prominent involvement of visuospatial functions, and a predominantly retrieval-type memory impairment. Behavioral symptoms such as hallucinations, apathy, and delusions are also frequent.

Although Alzheimer-type pathology, especially plaques, frequently accompany PDD, the main pathological correlate is Lewy body-type pathology in limbic and association cortices. The main biochemical deficit is loss of cholinergic markers, both in cholinergic nuclei as well as in the cerebral cortex. Therapeutic trials with cholinesterase inhibitors demonstrate moderate improvement in cognitive and behavioral symptoms. Based on these results, rivastigmine has been approved for treatment of PDD.

Murat Emre

Further reading

Emre M. Clinical features, pathophysiology and treatment of dementia associated with Parkinson's disease. In: Koller WC, Melamed E, eds. *Handbook of Neurology,* Vol. 83. Amsterdam: Elsevier BV, 2007: 401–20.

Emre M. Dementia associated with Parkinson's disease. *Lancet Neurol* 2003; **2**(4): 229–37.

Emre M. Dementia associated with Parkinson's disease: features and management. In: Jancovic J, Tolosa E, eds. *Parkinson's Disease and Movement Disorders,* 5th edn. Philadelphia: Lippincott, Williams & Wilkins, 2007: 152–60.

Case study 21

Case presentation

After being diagnosed with a colonic tumor, a 72-year-old Parkinson's disease (PD) patient was admitted for surgical removal of the tumor and a partial colectomy. His parkinsonian syndrome was characterized by predominant akinesia and rigidity, associated with gait and balance disturbances and mild cognitive deterioration. He was under treatment with levodopa/carbidopa 250/25 q.i.d. and quetiapine 25 mg at nighttime owing to the presence of occasional hallucinations and delusions. Levodopa afforded only partial relief of motor symptomatology, as it did not have a significant effect on axial symptomatology (speech, swallowing, posture, gait, and balance).

Upon recovery from anesthesia, the patient remained in a stuporous state with evident confusion, marked rigidity, and bradykinesia, requiring respiratory assistance owing to impaired ventilatory muscle function; swallowing was impaired and a nasoduodenal tube had to be placed. The patient was diaphoretic but afebrile, and had increased blood pressure (150/100) with preserved cardiac function. Laboratory results were unremarkable, except for an elevated leukocyte count and a threefold increase in creatine kinase (CK), which in this case could also be attributed to the surgery. The tube could not be used for the administration of medication as there was significant fluid yielding from it owing to the presence of a paralytic ileus.

I was called 36 h later to the intensive care unit (ICU), as the patient's condition was rapidly deteriorating. Faced with the impossibility of administering dopaminergic agents via the oral route or through the nasoduodenal tube, subcutaneous apomorphine was administered q.i.d. (5 mg) with a peripherally acting dopamine receptor blocker (domperidone) to prevent nausea and vomiting. Bowel sounds reappeared 24 h later; the paralytic ileus resolved, and the nasoduodenal tube stopped yielding fluid. Ventilatory assistance was stopped, and oral levodopa was started 48 h later. Administration of apomorphine not only allowed for recovery of intestinal transit, but improved respiratory function, and significantly reduced rigidity and bradykinesia, allowing for the withdrawal of the endotracheal tube as ventilatory function improved in parallel. The patient regained consciousness and became fully alert and oriented. A week later, he was discharged from the hospital to his home where he gradually recovered to a motor functional status that was somewhat worse than that in the preoperative period.

Discussion

This very brief clinical vignette is a clear example of some of the complications that can occur in the perioperative period when providing emergency care for PD patients, especially those who are elderly and have pre-existing axial motor and cognitive involvement. Such care requires the following points to be considered:
• decisions regarding surgery in a parkinsonian patient
• pharmacological management in the preoperative and the immediate postoperative period
• choosing the appropriate anesthesia in a PD patient
• respiratory and gastrointestinal factors influencing postoperative outcome in PD patients
• worsening of PD in the context of intercurrent disease.

Often we are confronted with PD patients who for different reasons have to undergo surgery and our opinion is sought regarding the risks involved in such situations. In cases where surgery is elective, we should carefully consider the risk/benefit ratio of the procedure given that complications in the perioperative period occur frequently in these patients. PD patients, especially elderly ones and those with predominantly axial involvement and cognitive deterioration, have increased chances of confusion, respiratory insufficiency, swallowing disorders, and reduced gastrointestinal motility in the postoperative period. Statistics show that 60% of hospitalized PD patients develop delirium or confusional states and that the inherent risk for its occurrence is eight times higher than in the control population.

The surgeon and anesthesiologist should also be aware that in PD patients, dysautonomia (including dysregulation of blood pressure in response to postural changes, propensity to develop arrhythmias, reduced gastric emptying and intestinal motility, etc.) is a frequent feature, and that respiratory abnormalities (both through impairment of central regulatory mechanisms and abnormal control and function of upper airway musculature) may be present and be aggravated by surgery.

An important contributing factor to postoperative outcome in PD patients is determined by the right choice of anesthesia. Anesthesiologists need to be instructed carefully on what drugs to avoid because of dangerous interactions or because they can aggravate the patient's motor functioning. Among the analgesics, meperidine or pethidine derivatives have potential interactions, especially in patients receiving selegiline, while morphine, as well as fentanyl and alfentanil, may aggravate rigidity. Volatile agents such as halothane carry the risk of inducing arrhythmias. Dopamine receptor blocking agents or antiemetics with significant central effects, such as metoclopramide, should also be avoided.

Regarding antiparkinson medication, the patient and carers should be made aware of the need to continue taking the medication until as close to the surgical procedure as possible. Furthermore, doctors and nurses have to be informed of the need to restart medication immediately after recovery from anesthesia, if possible via the oral route, or in cases where there is an impediment, through a nasogastric tube. As in the case of our patient, subcutaneous apomorphine can be used if it is necessary to bypass the gastrointestinal tract, which is frequently affected in the immediate postoperative period. The need for prompt restoration of dopaminergic stimulation is critical to the recovery of the patient as it helps in improving respiratory function, swallowing, proper clearing of pharyngolaryngeal and bronchial secretions, gastric emptying, intestinal motility, defecation, and urinary voiding.

Deterioration of motor function in PD is frequently observed in the presence of intercurrent disease or following surgical procedures. Surgery of the gastrointestinal tract is very frequently responsible for such deterioration, probably through a multifactorial mechanism including impairment of drug absorption. In our patient, worsening of PD was probably the result of these factors and drug withdrawal, as dopaminergic medication was not promptly reinstated. The ICU doctors were unaware of the possibility of using subcutaneous apomorphine as the most effective alternative in such cases.

Intercurrent illnesses, surgery, and drug withdrawal, alone or in combination as in the present case, carry an inherent risk of significant worsening of parkinsonism associated with additional clinical features. This syndrome has been recently reported in the literature as "parkinsonism–hyperpyrexia syndrome" (PHS). This term is used to refer to a clinical syndrome that is essentially identical to neuroleptic malignant syndrome (NMS) in the absence of exposure to neuroleptics, and often in the context of a reduction in dopamine agonist medications. This has also been referred to as an NMS-like syndrome and MS in PD. Clinically, symptoms include high fever, marked rigidity, disturbance of consciousness, autonomic dysfunction, and elevation of serum CK. Despite being observed frequently in the context of a reduction of dopaminergic therapy, they have been linked to other triggers such as intercurrent infections, surgery, heat exposure, and dehydration.

The term acute akinesia (AA) or acute akinetic crisis has also been used to describe a clinical syndrome of acute motor worsening in patients with PD. It is characterized by an akinetic state and transient unresponsiveness to antiparkinsonian medication without necessarily presenting with the additional features of PHS (fever, elevated CK, etc.). It has been also noted to occur in the context of infection, surgery, gastrointestinal disease, or changes in the therapeutic regime. All these syndromes are in fact probably the same clinical entity with variations in clinical presentation, in which the underlying pathogenesis is dopaminergic hypofunction in the nigrostriatal, hypothalamic and mesocortical systems owing to a variety of causes.

Our patient presented with almost all the clinical features (severe bradykinesia, increased rigidity, disturbance of consciousness, dysautonomia, a high leukocyte count and elevated CK) of PHS except for fever. It should be noted, however, that high CK in a patient having recently undergone surgery may not be attributed specifically to the syndrome. In addition, our patient did not show transient unresponsiveness to dopaminergic medication as the condition rapidly resolved with the administration of subcutaneous apomorphine.

This case underlies the need for careful evaluation of all the risk factors present in a PD patient undergoing surgery, and the crucial role that prompt restoration of dopaminergic stimulation has in avoiding postoperative complications and leading to a better outcome.

Final diagnosis: parkinsonism-hyperpyrexia syndrome.

Oscar S. Gershanik

Further reading

Frucht SJ. Movement disorder emergencies in the perioperative period. *Neurol Clin* 2004; **22**(2): 379–87.

Galvez-Jimenez N, Lang AE. The perioperative management of Parkinson's disease revisited. *Neurol Clin* 2004; **22**(2): 367–77.

Granner MA, Wooten GF. Neuroleptic malignant syndrome or parkinsonism hyperpyrexia syndrome. *Semin Neurol* 1991; **11**(3): 228–35.

Harada T, Mitsuoka K, Kumagai R *et al*. Clinical features of malignant syndrome in Parkinson's disease and related neurological disorders. *Parkinsonism Relat Disord* 2003; **9**: S15–S23.

Mizuno Y, Takubo H, Mizuta E *et al*. Malignant syndrome in Parkinson's disease: concept and review of the literature. *Parkinsonism Relat Disord* 2003; **9**: S3–9.

Nicholson G, Pereira AC, Hall GM. Parkinson's disease and anaesthesia. *Br J Anaesth* 2002; **89**(6): 904–16.

Onofrj M, Thomas A. Acute akinesia in Parkinson disease. *Neurology* 2005; **64**(7): 1162–9.

Takubo H, Harada T, Hashimoto T *et al*. A collaborative study on the malignant syndrome in Parkinson's disease and related disorders. *Parkinsonism Relat Disord* 2003; **9**: S31–41.

Case study 22

Case presentation

At 14 years of age, this right-handed accountant developed gait problems with his legs turning inward causing him to stumble, especially when running. About 10 years later, in his mid-twenties, he noticed clumsiness and stiffness of his right hand when performing fine finger movements and had difficulties with prolonged handwriting. Shortly thereafter, he started dragging his right leg. All of these symptoms were slowly progressive and began to involve the left hand side of his body over the course of the ensuing 5 years. At 30, the patient first experienced an intermittent tremor of his right hand that was mainly triggered by emotional stress. At this time, a diagnosis of Parkinson's disease (PD) was established by a neurologist who initiated treatment with levodopa (100 mg t.i.d.) and selegiline (5 mg in the morning). All of the patient's parkinsonian signs responded well to this therapy. His condition remained very slowly progressive, requiring little increase of his medication. At 42, now on a total dose daily of 600 mg of levodopa, the patient started to develop mild peak-dose dyskinesias but no motor fluctuations. Treatment trials with different dopamine agonists and amantadine were not tolerated by the patient owing to side effects.

His past medical history was unremarkable; in particular, there was no history of head trauma, meningoencephalitis, exposure to toxins, or intake of any drugs capable of inducing parkinsonism. He did not take any other regular medication, did not smoke, and drank alcohol only occasionally. He was divorced with two sons. The patient remained very active and continued to work full time. In addition, he engaged in different ambitious projects within the framework of a Parkinson's disease self-support group.

According to the patient, among his first-degree relatives, one of his sons showed possible mild signs of parkinsonism. In his more extended family, there was one maternal uncle with tremor, but no member with a diagnosis of definite Parkinson's disease.

On neurological examination at the age of 54, the patient showed generalized bradykinesia that was more pronounced on the right-hand side, and slight rigidity in both arms. There was an intermittent rest tremor of both arms that was brought out by performing serial sevens. The patient had no retropulsion and was rated as Hoehn and Yahr stage 2.5. His Unified Parkinson's Disease Rating Scale (UPDRS) III score (motor part, rated on medication) was 22 points (= moderate PD). In addition, he had mild choreiform dyskinesias of all four limbs. There were no cerebellar or pyramidal signs, no dysautonomia, or cognitive dysfunction. His Mini Mental State Examination score was 29/30. A magnetic resonance imaging scan was normal, as was routine laboratory testing. Transcranial ultrasound revealed marked bilateral hyperechogenicity of the substantia nigra. On fluorodopa positron emission tomography (PET), he showed a uniform pattern of decreased presynaptic fluorodopa uptake, most prominently in the posterior part of the putamen.

Differential diagnosis

Even in the absence of an obvious family history, a genetic form of parkinsonism should be considered in an individual with a very early age of disease onset. The patient developed unequivocal signs of parkinsonism in his midtwenties, preceded by a 10-year history of gait problems that were most likely owing to leg dystonia and probably the first manifestation of his disorder.

Mutations in the recessively inherited *Parkin* gene are by far the most common known cause of early-onset parkinsonism (EOP) and account for >70% of cases with an onset age below 30 years [1]. Although in many patients the clinical picture is indistinguishable from that of idiopathic PD, *Parkin* mutation carriers tend to have an overall earlier age of onset, slower disease progression, a more symmetrical onset, more frequently dystonia as the initial sign, hyperreflexia, and a tendency towards a better response to levodopa despite lower doses as compared to patients without *Parkin* mutations [2]. A practically identical clinical picture with a disease onset that is generally early has been associated with mutations in both the *PINK1* and *DJ1* genes that are also transmitted in a recessive fashion but that are much rarer than *Parkin* mutations. Finally, heterozygous mutations in the recently discovered *ATP13A2* gene have been reported in a few cases with clinically typical EOP [3]. The significance of this finding, however, will have to be evaluated in larger patient samples from different ethnic backgrounds. Homozygous and compound heterozygous mutations in *ATP13A2* had previously been identified in two families with a form of atypical parkinsonism termed Kufor–Rakeb syndrome [4].

With respect to dominant parkinsonism, mutations in α-synuclein can cause EOP, but mutations in this gene are exceedingly rare [5]. In contrast, pathological changes in the dominantly inherited *LRRK2* gene are a relatively frequent finding, but are usually associated with a later age of onset. (For review of genetic parkinsonism, see [6,7].)

Dystonia is frequent in EOP and sometimes its presenting sign. Conversely, parkinsonian signs occur in dopa-responsive dystonia (DRD), especially in later stages, and may even be the only finding in relatives of patients with clinically typical DRD [8]. Both conditions may have a similar age at onset and respond well to treatment with levodopa, thus adding mutations in the *GCH1* gene to the list of possible causes of parkinsonism. Of note, however, it is usually the DRD patients with a later age of onset who present with parkinsonism rather than dystonia.

In our patient, sequence and gene dosage analysis of the *Parkin* gene revealed compound heterozygous mutations on different alleles. One mutation was a known missense change (c.924C>T p.R275W) and the other one, a heterozygous deletion of exon 4 (delExon4).

Final diagnosis: *Parkin*-associated parkinsonism.

Discussion

Mutations in the *Parkin* gene have been shown in numerous families of different ethnic backgrounds worldwide [9]. The wide spectrum of *Parkin* mutations includes alterations in almost all exons. Importantly, >50% of the mutation carriers have exon rearrangements that, in the heterozygous state, are not detectable with qualitative screening methods [10,11]. Our patient was compound heterozygous for such an exon rearrangement (deletion of exon 4) and a missense change on the other *Parkin* allele. The R275W mutation is a relatively frequent finding among patients of European background, probably owing to a founder effect [9].

Although the overall clinical picture of our patient closely resembled that of idiopathic PD, he featured some of the clinical findings typically associated with *Parkin* parkinsonism, such as slow disease progression and a sustained response to antiparkinsonian medication after many years of treatment [2]. Since the patient's dystonic gait was probably the first manifestation of his disease, he would qualify as a case of juvenile parkinsonism (age of onset below 20 years). The identification of *Parkin* mutations in our patient further confirmed that mutations in this gene are a very common cause of parkinsonism in this age-of-onset group. The results of the additional investigations (transcranial ultrasound and PET) were typical of idiopathic PD and are not specific for genetic parkinsonism.

The family history of our patient was not strongly suggestive of a hereditary form of parkinsonism, as is often seen with recessively inherited parkinsonism in small families. It is possible that the report of tremor in a paternal uncle and signs of possible parkinsonism in the patient's son may be a clinical manifestation of heterozygous *Parkin* mutations. The role of heterozygous mutations as a susceptibility factor for parkinsonism, however, remains a matter of lively debate [12].

Taken together, our patient further highlights the following notions:

1 *Role and diagnosis of* Parkin-*associated parkinsonism*: *Parkin*-associated parkinsonism may mimic idiopathic PD at many levels, and a clear-cut diagnosis cannot be established solely on clinical grounds. *Parkin* mutations should be

considered as the first possible cause of juvenile and early-onset parkinsonism. The differential diagnosis includes mutations in *PINK1, DJ1, SNCA, LRRK2, GCHI* and possibly *ATP13A2*.

2 *Treatment and counseling of patients*: Although the individual clinical course cannot be predicted in a specific *Parkin* mutation carrier, the majority will progress more slowly and respond better to treatment than patients without mutations. Genetic testing of this gene is cumbersome and expensive and does not affect treatment. Furthermore, genetic counseling is complicated by the possible role of heterozygous mutations as susceptibility factors.

3 *General considerations*: Owing to its many similarities to idiopathic PD, our case raises the important question of a better definition and classification of idiopathic PD and other parkinsonian syndromes. *Parkin*-related parkinsonism may serve as a model for idiopathic PD, resulting in an improved understanding of shared pathogenetic pathways between *Parkin*-linked parkinsonism and idiopathic PD.

Christine Klein

References

1 Lucking CB, Durr A, Bonifati V *et al.* Association between early-onset Parkinson's disease and mutations in the parkin gene. French Parkinson's Disease Genetics Study Group. *N Engl J Med* 2000; **342**: 1560–7.

2 Lohmann E, Periquet M, Bonifati V *et al.* How much phenotypic variation can be attributed to parkin genotype? *Ann Neurol* 2003; **54**: 176–85.

3 Di Fonzo A, Chien HF, Socal M *et al.* ATP13A2 missense mutations in juvenile parkinsonism and young onset Parkinson disease. *Neurology* 2007; **68**: 1557–62.

4 Ramirez A, Heimbach A, Grundemann J *et al.* Hereditary parkinsonism with dementia is caused by mutations in ATP13A2, encoding a lysosomal type 5 P-type ATPase. *Nat Genet* 2006; **38**: 1184–91.

5 Berg D, Niwar M, Maass S *et al.* Alpha-synuclein and Parkinson's disease: implications from the screening of more than 1900 patients. *Mov Disord* 2005; **20**: 1191–4.

6 Klein C, Schlossmacher MG. Parkinson disease genetics: implications for neurological care. *Nature Clin Neurol* 2006; **2**: 136–46.

7 Klein C, Schlossmacher MG. Parkinson disease, 10 years after its genetic revolution. Multiple clues to a complex disorder. *Neurology* 2007; Aug 29 [Epub ahead of print].

8 Grimes DA, Bulman D, George-Hyslop PS, Lang AE. Inherited myoclonus-dystonia: evidence supporting genetic heterogeneity. *Mov Disord* 2001; **16**: 106–11.

9 Hedrich K, Eskelson C, Wilmot B *et al.* Distribution and origin of Parkin mutations: review and case studies. *Mov Disord* 2004; **19**: 1146–57.

10 Hedrich K, Kann M, Lanthaler AJ *et al.* The importance of gene dosage studies: mutational analysis of the parkin gene in early-onset parkinsonism. *Hum Mol Genet* 2001; **16**: 1649–56.

11 Djarmati A, Guzvić M, Grünewald A *et al.* Rapid and reliable detection of exon rearrangements in various movement disorders genes by multiplex ligation-dependent probe amplification. *Mov Disord* 2007; **22**(12): 1708–14.

12 Klein C, Lohmann-Hedrich K, Rogaeva E *et al.* Deciphering the role of heterozygous mutations in genes associated with parkinsonism. *Lancet Neurol* 2007; **6**: 652–62.

Case study 23

Case presentation

A 32-year-old woman presented with a 6-month history of right leg stiffness and intermittent slurred speech. There was a history of autoimmune hypothyroidism and a family history of thyroid disease and diabetes mellitus. The stiffness affected proximal and distal muscles of the right leg and interfered with voluntary movement of the leg. Muscle spasms were superimposed on the stiffness, further exacerbating the movement difficulties. Any external stimulus, particularly noise, touch, or an unexpected visual stimulus, resulted in a spasm. The spasms began with increasing stiffness in the quadriceps, spreading throughout the leg, straightening the leg then involving the trunk, limiting trunkal motion. These spasms could persist for several hours at a time and were accompanied by sweating, pallor, and severe lower back pain. Sudden spasms of the right leg had led to three falls. Over the following months, stiffness and spasms had spread to the left leg.

On examination the patient had "thick" speech with slow facial and tongue movements. There was a full range of eye movement. There was no myoclonus in response to tapping the face or upper chest. Muscle tone and strength in the upper limbs were within normal limits. The anterior abdominal muscles were rigid to palpation and there was paraspinal rigidity with prominent paraspinal muscle contours and an exaggerated lumbar lordosis. Passive rotation of the trunk was limited by rigidity. The right leg was rigid and passive movement was limited in all directions. Manipulation of the leg in the course of the examination and even lightly stroking the leg markedly increased rigidity of the trunk and leg.

Tendon reflexes in the upper limbs and left leg were brisk. When the right leg was not in spasm, tendon reflexes were also brisk. Plantar responses were flexor. Stimulation of the leg by touch or by tendon taps induced a small-amplitude myoclonic movement followed by a prolonged spasm with an increase in rigidity and extensor posturing of the leg. The amplitude of the initial myoclonic movement was restricted by the background rigidity. Sound induced a similar response. Stimulation of the unaffected left leg also produced an increase in tone in the right leg. Sensation was normal. She walked with stiff extended legs and reduced mobility of the lower trunk. Vitiligo was evident on the trunk.

Electrolytes, hematological, and biochemical screens were normal. Blood sugar levels ranged from 5 to 6.8 mmol/L (normal range 3.8–5.5 mmol/L). Antiglutamic acid decarboxylase antibody (antiGADab) titer was 67.5 u/mL (reference range 0–0.9). Thyroid stimulating hormone level was 4.9 mIU/L (0.5–3.7) and thyroxine was 16 pmol/L (10–25) consistent with early hypothyroidism. Thyroid peroxidase (TPO) antibodies were high (473 IU/mL; normal range < 50). Antiparietal cell antibodies were not detected. Cerebrospinal fluid contained four red blood cells, no white cells, 0.25 g/L protein (normal range 0.1–0.65 g/L) and 4.1 mmol/L glucose. Antinuclear and extractable nuclear antigen antibodies were not detected.

Magnetic resonance imaging (MRI) of the brain and spinal cord were normal. Mammography was normal. Electromyography (EMG) revealed continuous motor unit activity in muscles throughout the right leg and in the right paraspinal muscles despite attempted relaxation. Stimulation of the leg by touch or tendon taps induced a small-amplitude myoclonic movement followed by a prolonged increase in motor unit discharge. Surface EMG recordings from the right paraspinal, quadriceps femoris, and tibialis anterior muscles following (single pulse) stimulation of the right median, tibial (at the medial malleolus), and left tibial nerves elicited a stereotyped exteroceptive or cutaneomuscular reflex response in all muscles, beginning with one or two brief myoclonic potentials followed by a prolonged tonic response lasting > 1 s (Fig. 3.23.1). Magnetic stimulation of the brain elicited normal short latency "corticospinal" muscle action potentials followed by similar exteroceptive responses.

A slow infusion of diazepam (5 mg in 20 mL normal saline over 5 min) produced a dramatic reduction in stiffness and reflex spasms. Her speech improved and all movements of the trunk and legs, including walking, were much freer for the following 15 min.

Oral diazepam (15–30 mg) and baclofen (75 mg) daily improved the stimulus-induced spasms, but there was no lasting effect on leg and trunk rigidity and stiffness. Intravenous immunoglobulin at intervals of 3–4 months provided further benefit with a significant reduction in stiffness. This benefit began to wear off, however, around 3 months after each injection. She continues to receive infusions three to four times per month. Episodic spasms in response to unexpected stimuli, particularly sudden noise, emotional stress or surprise, continue to require additional doses of diazepam.

Differential diagnosis

The differential diagnosis of leg and trunk rigidity with an exaggerated lumbar lordosis [4] includes fibromyalgia and its variants, especially when there

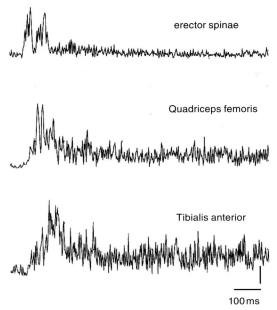

Figure 3.23.1 Rectified surface EMG recordings from the right erector spinae, quadriceps femoris, and tibialis anterior showing the response to electrical stimulation of the right median nerve (at the wrist). The average of five trials is shown. Stimuli were delivered at the start of the sweep. The response consists of one or two brief myoclonic potentials followed by a prolonged spasm lasting > 1 s. The latencies of the initial myoclonic bursts were 54, 65 and 81 ms respectively for the three muscles. A similar pattern of response (at different latencies) was elicited by stimulation at different sites. Vertical calibration bar represents 100 μV.

is accompanying pain; but continuous motor unit activity and rigidity are absent in contrast to stiff person syndrome (SPS). Axial dystonia, in which the abnormal trunkal posture settles during relaxation or when lying down, also needs to be excluded. The abnormal lumbar posturing of paraspinal myopathies with contracture persists during sleep and, in contrast to SPS, a reduced pattern of myopathic paraspinal motor units are found on EMG and fatty changes are evident on MRI of lumbar paraspinal muscles.

Symptoms commonly begin in one leg as in the present case and then spread to the trunk and opposite leg over months or years [4]. Follow-up over subsequent years reveals evolution to typical SPS [4] with leg and trunkal stiffness and rigidity. It is important to rule out structural or inflammatory spinal lesions as a cause of segmental rigidity and spasms (of one limb). The finding of enhanced exteroceptive reflexes is again of diagnostic value for SPS [4].

Continuous motor unit activity in trunkal and limb muscles with cocontraction of antagonist muscle groups may be evident in SPS, but in isolation this is not diagnostic as both may be found in dystonia, peripheral neuromuscular hyperexcitability syndromes, and spinal cord lesions with segmental rigidity.

Stimulus-induced spasms may also be an early presenting feature of SPS. Initially these may be very brief and without other neurological signs on examination. The transient nature of the stimulus (such as sudden noise, surprise, emotional stress) and the association with a brief spasm may escape notice, leading to a delay in diagnosis. In this situation and in the absence of trunkal or limb rigidity, a high degree of suspicion is required. When stimulus-induced spasms dominate the clinical picture with myoclonus, the term "jerking stiff man syndrome" has also been used [4]. In this situation, the enhanced exteroceptive reflexes are the neurophysiological basis for the spasms and myoclonus.

In our patient, dysarthria (which was due to stiffness of facial and lingual muscles and was dramatically relieved by intravenous diazepam) and the complaint of arm stiffness (though there were never any objective signs of upper limb involvement) were unusual features. The former raises the possibility of a related and overlapping condition: progressive encephalomyelitis with rigidity and myoclonus (PERM). The precise relationship of PERM to SPS is not clear [4]. Both may exhibit trunkal rigidity, enhanced exteroceptive reflexes, brainstem myoclonus, and antiGADabs. Cranial nerve abnormalities, especially ocular motor disturbances, bulbar palsies, and cerebellar ataxia, occur in PERM but not typical SPS. Despite these differences, there is overlap on pathological examination with perivascular lymphocytic cuffing and variable neuronal and interneuronal loss in the spinal cord in both clinical syndromes [5].

The onset of SPS in the upper limb also raises the possibility of a paraneoplastic origin, particularly in association with breast cancer [6]. Other paraneoplastic associations have also been described with antibodies to GAD and less commonly amphiphysin and gephyrin [6,7,8].

Final diagnosis: stiff person syndrome.

Discussion

The rarity of SPS adds to the difficulty of diagnosis in the early stages. By the time the present patient was referred for neurological review, however, there were many pointers to the diagnosis of SPS, particularly the combination of axial and lower limb rigidity with superimposed stimulus-induced spasms.

The expression "fluctuating muscular rigidity and spasm" in the original description of the "stiff man syndrome" by Moersch & Woltman emphasized the variability in severity of clinical signs and effect on functional capacity [1]. This remains a hallmark of the condition. The demonstration of enhanced exteroceptive reflexes as the neurophysiological basis for the stimulus-induced spasms is also characteristic of SPS [2].

Other helpful diagnostic features included the presence of antiGADabs. These are detected in 60–80% of cases and are the same antibodies found in type 1 diabetes mellitus (the titers are much higher in SPS) [3]. The presence of autoimmune endocrine disease (autoimmune thyroid disease is present in 10% of patients with SPS) was an additional clue to SPS [3,4].

Treatment

A variety of drugs have been reported to be of value in treating SPS. The most useful are γ-aminobutyric acid (GABA) agonists such as baclofen and diazepam in reducing spasms. A variety of anticonvulsants that modulate GABA transmission have also been shown to be of value in small series and case reports, but there have been no systematic trials into their efficacy. The demonstration of antiGADabs in SPS has raised the question of an autoimmune basis for the condition and prompted trials of immune modulatory therapies. Methyl prednisolone, plasma exchange, immunosuppression, and intravenous immunoglobulin (IVIG) have all been tried. To date the only controlled trial evidence of benefit is for the use of IVIG [9].

Philip D. Thompson

References

1 Moersch FP, Woltman HW. Progressive fluctuating muscular rigidity and spasm (stiff-man syndrome): report of a case and some observations in 13 other cases. *Mayo Clin Proc* 1956; **31**: 421–7.

2 Meinck HM, Ricker K, Conrad B. The stiff man syndrome: new pathophysiological aspects from abnormal exteroceptive reflexes and the response to clomipramine, clonidine, and tizanidine. *J Neurol Neurosurg Psychiatry* 1984; **47**: 280–7.

3 Solimena M, Folli F, Aparisi R, Pozza G, De Camilli P. Autoantibodies to GABAergic neurons and pancreatic beta cells in stiff-man syndrome. *N Engl J Med* 1990; **322**: 1555–60.

4 Meinck HM, Thompson PD. The stiff man syndrome and related conditions. *Mov Disord* 2002; **17**: 853–66.

5 Warren JD, Scott G, Blumbergs PC, Thompson PD. Pathological evidence of encephalomyelitis in the stiff man syndrome with anti GAD antibodies. *J Clin Neurosci* 2002; **9**: 328–9.

6 Folli F, Solimena M, Cofiell R *et al.* Autoantibodies to a 128-kd synaptic protein in three women with the stiff-man syndrome and breast cancer. *N Engl J Med* 1993; **328**: 546–51.

7 Dropcho EJ. Antiamphiphysin antibodies with small-cell lung carcinoma and paraneoplastic encephalomyelitis. *Ann Neurol* 1996; **39**: 659–67.

8 Butler HM, Hatashi A, Ohkoshi N *et al.* Autoimmunity to gephyrin in stiff-man syndrome. *Neuron* 2000; **26**: 307–12.

9 Dalakas MC, Fujii M, Li M, Lufti B, Kyhos J, McElroy B. High dose intravenous immunoglobulin for stiff person syndrome. *N Engl J Med* 2001; **345**: 1870–6.

Case study 24

Case presentation

A 52-year-old right-handed man was referred to the Neurology Clinic because of intermittent tremor and clumsiness of the left arm over the preceding year.

The patient had been well until 2 years ago, when he developed slowly progressive gait disturbance and stiffness in his left leg. He was examined by a neurologist 6 months after the onset of these symptoms. Magnetic resonance imaging of the brain and entire spinal cord, cerebrospinal fluid examination, and routine blood and urine tests were all normal. A diagnosis of lower limb spasticity of unknown cause was made. He was treated with baclofen and diazepam without any improvement. He therefore stopped taking these medications. About 4 months later he developed slowness and clumsiness of his left hand. This was followed by an intermittent rest tremor of the same hand that was aggravated by emotional distress. He was not taking any medications at that time.

His general health had always been good. He denied history of encephalitis, meningitis, head trauma, exposure to industrial toxins, psychotropic medications, or illicit drug usage. He denied depression, anxiety, and difficulties with sleep or balance.

The patient was the oldest of three siblings; the two younger sisters were healthy. His father had died of a heart attack at 48 years of age. His mother had undergone mastectomy at 61 years of age for breast carcinoma. She died 5 years later. The paternal grandmother had suffered from tremor and progressive slowness of movements during the last decade of her life. The patient was unaware of his grandmother's diagnosis, however, and her medical records were not available for inspection. A maternal aunt had been diagnosed with Parkinson's disease (PD) at 63 years of age. The patient was not aware of any neurological disease in his parents or any other relatives.

General physical and cranial nerve examinations in the patient were normal. Mental status was normal, with a Mini Mental Status Examination score of 29/30. Speech was normal. He had mild hypomimia. His resting tremor was intermittent, with a frequency of about 5 Hz and a moderate amplitude affecting his left hand. No postural or action tremor was visible. A mild rigidity was present in his left extremities, with dystonic posturing of the left foot that was held in plantar flexion and inversion at the ankle. Mild to moderate bradykinesia was noted in the left hand, but none on the right side. No muscle weakness or sensory abnormality was identified. His gait was somewhat slow and shuffling. Deep-tendon reflexes were minimally exaggerated but symmetrical, and plantar responses were flexor. No signs of autonomic dysfunction were present. Diagnostic procedures were performed.

Differential diagnosis

The movement disorder of this patient is characterized by left-sided parkinsonism with resting tremor, rigidity, and bradykinesia. There was also dystonia affecting his left foot. The combination of parkinsonism and dystonia can occur in a number of movement disorders, including sporadic PD. Some dystonias (e.g. painful foot dystonias) are frequent in PD and can occur as a result of antiparkinsonian treatment. Dystonia can also be observed in untreated PD patients, however, although this is less common. When dystonia is present in PD prior to the initiation of levodopa therapy, it usually involves the lower extremities and is located ipsilateral to the parkinsonian symptomatology. As in our patient, other symptoms of PD normally emerge shortly after the onset of dystonia.

The patient's family history of parkinsonism provides diagnostic clues. His father died at a young age; therefore, the mode of inheritance could be autosomal dominant, possibly with reduced penetrance. In the past few years, several genetic mutations have been identified in familial parkinsonism, including in a number of patients with a clinical presentation indistinguishable from sporadic PD. The first gene identified for autosomal dominantly inherited parkinsonism (PARK1) was α-*synuclein* [1]. Three missense mutations, as well as multiplications of the complete wild-type gene, have been described. Clinically, most studied patients with α-*synuclein* mutations showed typical features of parkinsonism, including the cardinal features and a positive response to levodopa treatment. Some mutation carriers presented a broader phenotype with prominent dementia, orthostatic hypotension, and myoclonus [2]. Compared with sporadic PD cases, most α-*synuclein* mutation carriers present with a relatively early disease onset, and disease progression is usually faster. Mutations in this gene are very rare, and genetic testing for this gene is not commercially available.

Recently, a large number of mutations have been found in the *leucine-rich repeat kinase 2* (*LRRK2*) gene (PARK8) both in autosomal-dominant parkinsonism and patients with seemingly sporadic disease [3,4]. Clinically, most individuals with *LRRK2* mutations have symptoms compatible with sporadic late-onset PD. The patients have asymmetric parkinsonism and the most common initial presentation has been bradykinesia and unilateral resting tremor. Response to levodopa therapy has been reported as good, and motor complications have developed in half the patients receiving treatment [5]. Few of the individuals presented with atypical symptoms, although a few patients have presented with a supranuclear gaze palsy, amyotrophy, and dementia [3]. Levodopa-responsive foot dystonia has been described as the initial symptom in several patients.

Dystonia at disease onset is relatively frequent in parkinsonism associated with mutations in the *Parkin* gene. The disease course of *Parkin* disease is relatively benign with slow disease progression, sleep benefit and good response to levodopa, but complicated with early motor fluctuations and development of dyskinesias. *Parkin* mutations were first identified in early-onset autosomal recessive parkinsonism, and numerous mutations (> 100), including exonic deletions, insertions, and point mutations, have now been found in patients of all ethnic backgrounds. Mutations in this gene are common in early-onset parkinsonism. The chance of finding *Parkin* mutations in a patient with PD, however, decreases significantly with increased age at onset. *Parkin* mutations are rare in patients with late-onset disease (> 50 years) [6]. Commercial testing for *Parkin* mutations with complete gene sequencing and gene-dose assessment is available.

The combination of parkinsonism and dystonia can also occur in primary dystonias, a group of disorders increasingly recognized as being inherited. Idiopathic torsion dystonia (DYT1) is a generalized form of dystonia inherited as an autosomal dominant trait with reduced penetrance. *DYT1* mutations account for 90% of childhood-onset dystonia in Ashkenazi Jews and 50% in other populations, with a penetrance of 30%. The onset of disease symptoms, however, generally occurs before 26 years of age [7]. Genetic testing for *DYT1* gene is commercially available.

Dopa-responsive dystonia (DYT5) is characterized by progressive dystonia starting in one extremity and concurrent or subsequent parkinsonism with a dramatic response to levodopa. Disease onset is usually in childhood or adolescence, but adult-onset forms do exist. Parkinsonism is more frequent in patients with later disease onset. In most families this disorder is inherited as an autosomal-dominant trait caused by mutations in the gene for GTP cyclohydrolase 1, an enzyme in tetrahydrobiopterin synthesis [8]. Tetrahydrobiopterin is an essential cofactor for tyrosine hydroxylase, the rate-limiting enzyme for dopamine synthesis, with a resulting dopamine deficiency that explains the symptoms.

In this patient there was a family history of parkinsonism, but no family history of dystonia. Thus a form of familial parkinsonism clinically resembling sporadic PD is most likely. Dopa-responsive dystonia cannot be excluded, however, based on the available clinical information of the affected relatives. Therapeutic response to dopaminergic treatment would be an important diagnostic test. Dopa-responsive dystonia normally has a dramatic response to small doses of levodopa within a few days, while neurodegenerative parkinsonism has a less dramatic response and could require higher doses of levo-dopa. Dopamine transporter (DAT) imaging using single photon emission computed tomography (SPECT) or positron emission tomography (PET) may be useful in separating dopa-responsive dystonia, a disorder with preserved nigrostriatal projections, from neurodegenerative forms of familial parkinsonism with reduced striatal tracer uptake.

Final diagnosis: Autosomal-dominant parkinsonism caused by a 6055G>A mutation (Gly2019Ser) in the *LRRK2* gene.

Discussion

In this patient, SPECT imaging after injection of ^{123}I-FP-CIT showed bilaterally reduced tracer uptake in the putamen (Fig. 3.24.1). The reduction was more pronounced on the right side and tracer uptake in the caudate nuclei was less affected. These findings are typical for sporadic PD and similar results have been obtained in patients with familial parkinsonism. Abnormal DAT imaging excludes dopa-responsive dystonia as a diagnosis. Pramipexol, a dopamine agonist, was started and slowly increased up to a dose of 0.7 mg t.i.d. The patient reported a marked improvement in his symptoms. The dystonic posture of the left leg disappeared completely and the bradykinesia improved. The patient's tremor decreased, but was still present in stressful situations.

Genetic testing of the most common *LRRK2* mutations was performed and the patient was heterozygous for a 6055G>A mutation in exon 41, leading to a Gly2019Ser amino acid substitution of the Lrrk2 protein sequence. The *LRRK2* gene is a large gene with 51 exons and encodes a protein kinase with largely unknown function. Since the discovery of the *LRRK2* gene in 2004, a large number of variants have been identified in this gene, but there are

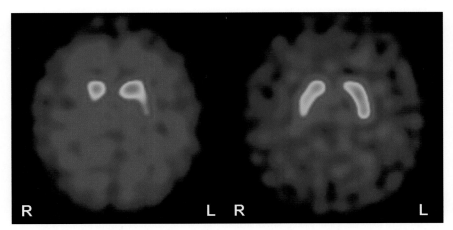

Figure 3.24.1 SPECT imaging with ^{123}I-FP-CIT; left, the patient; right, the normal control subject. Tracer uptake in the putamen is bilaterally reduced with a more pronounced reduction on the right side. Tracer uptake in the caudate nuclei is less affected.

only six genetically proven pathogenic mutations. These mutations, including Gly2019Ser, are linked with disease in families and clearly segregate with disease. The Gly2019Ser mutation is a relatively frequent cause of parkinsonism, with mutation frequencies varying between 0.5% and 5% in most sporadic PD populations [9].

The presented case highlights several features of *LRRK2*-associated disease. In *LRRK2*-associated parkinsonism the age of onset is variable, but most patients develop parkinsonian symptoms after the age of 50 years. The penetrance of *LRRK2* mutations is reduced and age-dependent, increasing from 17% at age 50 years to 85% at age 70 years [10]. Mutations are therefore frequently found in patients without a clear autosomal-dominant family history of parkinsonsim.

Several hundred patients with the *LRRK2* Gly2019Ser mutation have been reported in the literature, and few of these patients had any atypical symptoms. Dementia, autonomic dysfunction, and other neurologic signs do not seem to be more frequent than in patients with sporadic PD [11]. Also DAT imaging has been reported to be comparable to the findings in sporadic disease [12]. On neuropathological examination, the mutation is associated with Lewy body disease [13]. Autosomal dominant parkinsonism associated with the *LRRK2* Gly2019Ser mutation can therefore be both clinically and pathologically indistinuguishable from sporadic PD. Whether dystonia is more frequent in *LRRK2*-associated parkinsonism than sporadic PD has so far not been studied in detail.

Mathias Toft, Zbigniew K. Wszolek

References

1 Polymeropoulos MH, Lavedan C, Leroy E *et al*. Mutation in the alpha-synuclein gene identified in families with Parkinson's disease. *Science* 1997; **276**: 2045–7.

2 Spira PJ, Sharpe DM, Halliday G, Cavanagh J, Nicholson GA. Clinical and pathological features of a parkinsonian syndrome in a family with an Ala53Thr alpha-synuclein mutation. *Ann Neurol* 2001; **49**: 313–19.

3 Zimprich A, Biskup S, Leitner P *et al*. Mutations in *LRRK2* cause autosomal-dominant parkinsonism with pleomorphic pathology. *Neuron* 2004; **44**: 601–7.

4 Paisan-Ruiz C, Jain S, Evans EW *et al*. Cloning of the gene containing mutations that cause PARK8-linked Parkinson's disease. *Neuron* 2004; **44**: 595–600.

5 Aasly JO, Toft M, Fernandez-Mata I *et al*. Clinical features of *LRRK2*-associated Parkinson's disease in central Norway. *Ann Neurol* 2005; **57**: 762–5.

6 Gosal D, Ross OA, Toft M. Parkinson's disease: the genetics of a heterogeneous disorder. *Eur J Neurol* 2006; **13**: 616–27.

7 de Carvalho Aguiar PM, Ozelius LJ. Classification and genetics of dystonia. *Lancet Neurol* 2002; **1**: 316–25.

8 Segawa M, Nomura Y, Nishiyama N. Autosomal dominant guanosine triphosphate cyclohydrolase I deficiency (Segawa disease). *Ann Neurol* 2003; **54**(Suppl 6): S32–45.

9 Farrer MJ. Genetics of Parkinson disease: paradigm shifts and future prospects. *Nat Rev Genet* 2006; **7**: 306–18.

10 Kachergus J, Mata IF, Hulihan M *et al.* Identification of a novel *LRRK2* mutation linked to autosomal dominant parkinsonism: evidence of a common founder across European populations. *Am J Hum Genet* 2005; **76**: 672–80.

11 Nichols WC, Pankratz N, Hernandez D *et al.* Genetic screening for a single common *LRRK2* mutation in familial Parkinson's disease. *Lancet* 2005; **365**: 410–12.

12 Isaias IU, Benti R, Goldwurm S *et al.* Striatal dopamine transporter binding in Parkinson's disease associated with the *LRRK2* Gly2019Ser mutation. *Mov Disord* 2006; **21**: 1144–7.

13 Ross OA, Toft M, Whittle AJ *et al.* Lrrk2 and Lewy body disease. *Ann Neurol* 2006; **59**: 388–93.

Case study 25

Case presentation

A 65-year-old right-handed surgeon presented for evaluation of a 4-year history of progressive left-sided clumsiness and stiffness. He had initially noted difficulties coordinating the movements of his left hand when putting on his surgical gloves or when using his surgical instruments, and this had forced his early retirement. He had also developed a tendency to catch the toes of his left foot when climbing stairs. In the year prior to his evaluation, he had begun having difficulty using his right hand, and his left arm had begun to posture involuntarily. He had lost the ability to write and could no longer read, principally because of difficulty moving his eyes across the page. He was tripping frequently and occasionally falling. His intellectual abilities had not declined; however, he needed help to dress, eat, shave, and shower. He stated that it was as if he had forgotten how to perform these and other "automatic" activities previously taken for granted.

On our initial evaluation, the patient's left arm was held in a dystonic posture, flexed at the elbow, wrist and fingers. The right hand tended to levitate involuntary towards the face. Occasionally, the right shoulder would elevate and the left foot would intort. Mental status testing was normal, apart from marked impairment of clock drawing and figure copying. Cranial nerve examination revealed slowed tongue movements, mild oral-buccal apraxia, and minor difficulty initiating voluntary saccades. Motor examination demonstrated appendicular rigidity, slowed hand and finger movements, and an action tremor, all worse on the left. The patient was unable to carry out purposeful movements with the left upper limb, and made hand-as-object apraxic errors on the right. Gait was mildly apraxic. The remainder of the examination was unremarkable.

Computed tomography revealed moderate atrophy of the posterior fossa structures and mild cortical atrophy, more pronounced on the right hemisphere than on the left. Neuropsychological testing suggested frontotemporal lobe dysfunction. A limited metabolic workup was unremarkable.

The patient presented with a chronic, progressive neurological disorder, characterized by early asymmetric rigidity, dystonia, arm levitation, and apraxia which ultimately came to dominate the clinical picture. As the patient's disease progressed, he developed a variety of additional features, including cortical sensory loss, hemisensory neglect, and myoclonus. The disease process therefore localizes to both cortex and basal ganglia. Symptoms suggestive of cortical involvement are apraxia, cortical sensory loss, hemisensory neglect, and myoclonus; the features typically, although not exclusively [1], referable to basal ganglia dysfunction are represented by bradykinesia, dystonia, and tremor.

Differential diagnosis

The patient's age and the slow time course of his disease suggest a neurodegenerative condition. In the broadest sense, his presentation can be characterized as an atypical parkinsonism or a "Parkinson plus" syndrome. Its complexity and especially the features suggesting focal and asymmetric cortical involvement, however, justify the more specific classification of "corticobasal syndrome" (CBS). The core clinical features of CBS are progressive asymmetric rigidity and apraxia. Numerous additional findings suggestive of either cortical or basal ganglia pathology may be present. CBS was once thought relatively specific for a pathological diagnosis of corticobasal degeneration (CBD), but as awareness of the condition has grown, so too has our understanding that a variety of pathologies producing focal and asymmetric topographies of neurodegeneration can present with the core clinical features of the syndrome [1–3] (Table 3.25.1).

Conversely, it has become equally clear that pathologically confirmed CBD may present clinically with features more typical of other neurodegenerative conditions, including a primary progressive aphasia, frontotemporal dementia, a posterior cortical atrophy syndrome, progressive hemiparesis, and a pure progressive apraxia [4–6]. These observations highlight an important principle in the conceptualization of neurodegenerative syndromes: the clinical presentation of a patient depends on the topography of the brain targeted by the pathologic process rather than the pathology itself.

Final diagnosis: corticobasal degeneration.

Discussion

At the time of the patient's initial evaluation in our clinic in the early 1980s, his presentation was felt to be most consistent with CBD. Four years later, this diagnosis was confirmed on autopsy.

CBD is a rare disease: its prevalence has been estimated in one study to be 4.9–7.3 per 100 000, as compared to 100–250 per 100 000 for PD [7]. This is at best a tenuous estimate, however, as the proportion of patients presenting with the classical syndrome vs. one of the alternative manifestations remains

Table 3.25.1 More common causes of the corticobasal syndrome (CBS)

Pathology	Typical clinical features[a]
Corticobasal degeneration	Apraxia, dystonia, asymmetric rigidity Cortical findings: sensory loss, myoclonus, dementia Alien limb: uncommon at presentation; develops in 50%
Progressive supranuclear palsy	Early vertical supranuclear gaze palsy (but can be absent in early or atypical disease) Rigidity: typically axial and symmetric rather than appendicular and asymmetric Early falls Wide-eyed severely masked facies
Dementia with Lewy bodies	Early dementia, fluctuations Psychosis, hallucinations
Pick's disease	Frontotemporal dementia syndrome, personality change Often in younger patient
Vascular parkinsonism	Stepwise progression is typical MRI: multiple infarcts
Alzheimer's disease	Early "cortical" dementia
Frontotemporal dementia with parkinsonism-17	Family history of parkinsonism or dementia (typically frontotemporal) including CBS Can occur in younger patient
Progranulin mutations	Family history of parkinsonism or dementia (typically frontotemporal) including CBS Can occur in younger patient
Neurofilament inclusion body disease	Young patient (under age 50) Rapid course 2.5–5 years
Dementia with ubiquitin-positive inclusions (with and without motor neuron disease)	Rapidly progressive disease Typically frontotemporal dementia
Creutzfeldt–Jakob disease	Rapid progression < 2 years (rare cases with more prolonged course reported) Dementia typically pronounced and early MRI/Flair and diffusion-weighted images: increased signal in basal ganglia and cortical rim Electroencephalogram: periodic sharp wave complexes

[a] These disorders may present with all of the classical features of CBS. Their "Typical Clinical Features" usually assist us in differentiating them one from another and from corticobasal degeneration; however, at the onset of disease and even throughout much of its course, these features may not always be evident.

unknown. The classical syndrome typically presents in the sixth to eighth decades of life, with some manifestation of progressive asymmetric rigidity and apraxia, most commonly involving a hand, and occasionally with additional features such as stimulus-induced or action myoclonus. As the disease progresses, a mixture of movement disorders develops, including dystonia (typically involving the distal limbs), myoclonus, postural and action tremor, alien limb phenomena, and parkinsonism. The latter may begin in a markedly asymmetric manner, but typically progresses to produce postural instability and falls, as well as dysarthria and dysphagia.

Apraxia is almost universal during the course of CBD. The spectrum includes limb-kinetic apraxia, often a very early feature, and ideomotor and ideational apraxia, which may evolve later in the disease. Alien limb phenomenon is reported in up to 50% of patients, with the most common form likely being utilization behavior – compulsive groping and manipulation of objects. More purposeful movements such as intermanual conflict are less frequently seen. Levitation of a limb, sometimes called the posterior variant of alien limb, also occurs but is not specific for CBD. Cortical sensory loss is another important feature of the disorder. Oculomotor impairment is common and may present with an ocular gaze apraxia which may then evolve to a supranuclear gaze palsy, often equal in vertical and horizontal vectors. Isolated apraxia of speech or non-fluent aphasia may be the initial manifestations of the disorder. Finally, cognitive dysfunction is now recognized as a common feature of CBD. It may also dominate the presentation early in the disease course, to the point where patients are initially classified as having a frontotemporal dementia.

In the absence of validated diagnostic criteria and specific biomarkers for CBD, accurate antemortem diagnosis remains challenging [8]. Results of routine blood and cerebrospinal fluid analysis are typically normal. No imaging features are specific to the diagnosis, as current modalities delineate only the topography of the brain affected by the pathology rather than specific features of the pathology itself. Anatomical and functional imaging studies can nonetheless support a diagnosis of CBD by revealing asymmetric cortical frontoparietal and subcortical disturbances, more prominent contralateral to the side of the body most affected clinically.

Mean survival is 8 years after symptom onset. The disease progresses to bilateral involvement and eventually produces a bed-bound state, with death typically resulting from aspiration pneumonia or urosepsis. Early bilateral bradykinesia or frontal dementia predict a shorter survival [9]. The disorder is sporadic, but a genetic predisposition is suggested by rare reports of similarly affected relatives and an association with certain haplotypes of the microtubule-associated protein tau (*MAPT*) gene.

CBD is classified as a tauopathy in which isoforms of the protein containing 4 repeats of a microtubule binding domain predominate. Other members of this class of neurodegenerative diseases include progressive supranuclear palsy and frontotemporal dementia with parkinsonism linked to chromosome 17. Gross pathological features of CBD include asymmetric frontoparietal cortical and subcortical atrophy and ventricular dilatation. Microscopic changes include neuronal loss and gliosis in a wide cortical and subcortical distribution, including the substantia nigra where basophilic "corticobasal inclusions" may also be found. Immunohistochemistry is now required for diagnosis, and should demonstrate prominent tau-positive neuropil threads and astrocytic plaques. Swollen "ballooned" achromatic neurons identical to Pick cells are a common but non-specific feature, as are "coiled bodies" in oligodendrocytes.

No therapy alters disease progression, and none markedly improves symptoms. Management therefore consists primarily of physical, occupational and speech therapies, as well as judicious use of medications for all the usual complications of atypical parkinsonism. A clear response to levodopa is rare and lack of improvement with a robust trial of levodopa therapy above 900 mg per day is in fact one of the diagnostic features of this and other Parkinson-plus disorders.

Despite clinical and pathological differences between the four repeat tauopathies, advances in the management of any one of these conditions will likely enhance our understanding of the others. Current studies are attempting to define reliable biomarkers that may provide insight into the pathogenesis of these disorders, facilitate the development and evaluation of drugs to treat them, and assist in their early diagnosis when the latter become available.

Thomas D.L. Steeves, Anthony E. Lang

References

1 Boeve BF, Maraganore DM, Parisi JE *et al.* Pathologic heterogeneity in clinically diagnosed corticobasal degeneration. *Neurology* 1999; **53**: 795–800.
2 Lang AE, Bergeron C, Pollanen MS, Ashby P. Parietal Pick's disease mimicking cortical-basal ganglionic degeneration. *Neurology* 1994; **44**: 1436–40.
3 Bergeron C, Pollanen MS, Weyer L, Black SE, Lang AE. Unusual clinical presentations of cortical-basal ganglionic degeneration. *Ann Neurol* 1996; **40**: 893–900.
4 Bhatia KP, Lee MS, Rinne JO *et al.* Corticobasal degeneration look-alikes. *Adv Neurol* 2000; **82**: 169–82.
5 Kertesz A, Martinez-Lage P, Davidson W, Munoz DG. The corticobasal degeneration syndrome overlaps progressive aphasia and frontotemporal dementia. *Neurology* 2000; **55**: 1368–75.
6 Caselli RJ, Jack CR, Jr. Asymmetric cortical degeneration syndromes. A proposed clinical classification. *Arch Neurol* 1992; **49**: 770–80.
7 Togasaki DM, Tanner CM. Epidemiologic aspects. *Adv Neurol* 2000; **82**: 53–9.
8 Hughes AJ, Daniel SE, Ben-Shlomo Y, Lees AJ. The accuracy of diagnosis of parkinsonian syndromes in a specialist movement disorder service. *Brain* 2002; **125**: 861–70.
9 Wenning GK, Litvan I, Jankovic J *et al.* Natural history and survival of 14 patients with corticobasal degeneration confirmed at postmortem examination. *J Neurol Neurosurg Psychiatry* 1998; **64**: 184–9.

3   Case studies—diagnostic index

1	Parkinson's disease (PD) with a history of premotor symptoms	Eduardo Tolosa, Carles Gaig, Yaroslau Compta, Alex Iranzo, Francesc Valldeoriola
2	Early PD (utility of DAT SPECT imaging)	Heike Stockner, Werner Poewe
3	Wilson's disease	Jean-Marc Trocello, France Woimant
4	Spinocerebellar ataxia (SCA2 mimicking Parkinson's disease)	Perrine Charles, Alexandra Dürr, Alexis Brice
5	PD-mimicking Huntington disease	André R. Troiano, Leorah Freeman, Alexandra Dürr
6	Early PD (differential diagnosis of subtle features of parkinsonism)	Jayne R. Wilkinson, Matthew B. Stern
7	Multiple system atrophy	Wassilios Meissner, François Tison
8	Progressive supranuclear palsy	Irene Litvan
9	Fluctuations in motor performance: wearing-off	Marcus M. Unger, Wolfgang H. Oertel
10	Diphasic dyskinesia	Fabrizio Stocchi
11	End-of-dose dyskinesia	Philippe Damier
12	PD-related depression	Matthias R. Lemke
13	PD with indication for deep brain stimulation	Pierre Pollak
14	Mild cognitive impairment in PD	Bruno Dubois, Virginie Czernecki
15	Dementia with Lewy bodies	Terry McClain, Robert A. Hauser
16	Tremulous PD versus essential tremor	Georg H. Kägi, Kailash P. Bhatia
17	Vascular parkinsonism	Ruth Djaldetti, Eldad Melamed
18	Treatment-related impulse control disorder in PD	Daniel Weintraub

19	Gaucher disease complicated by parkinsonism	Frédéric Sedel
20	PD with dementia	Murat Emre
21	Emergency care: parkinsonism-hyperpyrexia syndrome	Oscar S. Gershanik
22	*Parkin*-associated parkinsonism	Christine Klein
23	Stiff person syndrome	Philip D. Thompson
24	Autosomal-dominant parkinsonism (*LRRK2* mutation)	Mathias Toft, Zbigniew K. Wszolek
25	Corticobasal degeneration	Thomas D.L. Steeves, Anthony E. Lang